STRESSED OUT ABOUT NURSING SCHOOL!

STRESSED OUT ABOUT NURSING SCHOOL!

An Insider's Guide to Success

Stephanie Thibeault

BANDIDO
BOOKS

Includes references and index. Orlando, Florida 2001

ISBN 1-929693-16-8

Cartoon illustration by Carl Elbing Jr.
Art direction and design by David Morales.
Printed in the United States of America.

To keep abreast of changes, additions and new products, please visit us at *www.bandidobooks.com* or contact us via email at *publish@bandidobooks.com* or by postal service at:

Bandido Books
9806 Heaton Court
Orlando, FL 32817

Happy Nursing!

Nursing at Clinical Speed!

For order information call our Toll-Free Hotline at 1-877-814-6824 PIN 1174

Reviewers

Patricia C. Bennett RN, MSN
Assistant Professor
Molloy College
Rockville Centre, New York

Monica Hidaji Student Nurse
Southwest Tennessee Community College
Memphis, Tennessee

Sandy Martin LPN, Student Nurse
Lehigh Carbon Community College
Schnecksville, Pennsylvania

Teri Ourada Student Nurse
Austin Peay State University
Clarksville, Tennessee

Mary Margaret Richardson EdD, RN, CNS
Associate Dean
Valdosta State University
Valdosta, Georgia

Sharon Trussell LPN, Student Nurse
Wallace State Community College
Hanceville Alabama

About the Author

Stephanie Thibeault is a second-career nursing student working towards her goal to become a hospice nurse practitioner. She has over 10 years experience in administration and human resources, and has devoted significant time to volunteer work in the social service and healthcare sectors. She is the developer of an award-winning website for nursing students, The Student Nurse Forum, and publishes a monthly journal, The Student Nurse Advisor. Stephanie lives in Kansas City with her two children, Anthony and Emma.

Acknowledgements

I would like to acknowledge the following individuals who generously shared their experiences and advice for use in this book: Patricia Bennett, Cynthia Schudel, Sandy Martin, Victor and Kathy Fernandez, Louise Komorek, Emily Horne, Patricia Erickson, Sally Villasenor, Vickie Milazzo, and Leigh Owen. I would also like to express my enormous gratitude and appreciation for the expert guidance, advice and editing skills of Martin Schiavenato, and the wonderful graphic design skills of David Morales, who made this book look fantastic. Finally, I would like to thank my parents for their support and encouragement, which has given me the wings to fly as I follow my dreams.

Dedication

This book is dedicated to my two children, Anthony and Emma, who inspire me everyday.

Table of Contents

Part Three: Beyond the Classroom

How to Use this Book

What if there was a book that explained complex nursing topics in an easy to understand manner, and in an accessible format? That's the premise behind the *Stressed Out About...Series*. Solid references with a bit of a sense of humor and the understanding that a lighthearted approach to learning makes the whole thing more enjoyable.

To help you navigate through the book, you will find the following *Icons* highlighting a particular passage:

Ask

This icon directs you to seek or search further information from an individual or organization.

Don't Forget

A little reminder about something of importance.

Don't Panic

Take a deep breath and relax, here is a little reassurance.

Fact

Highlights a statistic or "truth."

Tip

A bit of "inside information," a hint, or helpful advice.

Watch Out

"Words to the wise," this is a warning.

bandidobooks.com

This icon refers you to our Web Site where you may find further information on the topic.

Happy Nursing! Now you're ready to get started...

Introduction

So You Want to Be a Nurse...

The road to becoming a nurse is not easy - you won't find any sugarcoating in this book. As a matter of fact, *nursing* is not easy - it takes a special person to be a nurse. But it IS worth it and you can do it!

This book was written to help you on your path to becoming a nurse. Think of it as your personal guidebook. Offering valuable insight and advice every step of the way, this book will support and encourage you as you follow your dream.

Stressed Out About Nursing School: An Insider's Guide to Success will walk you through everything you need to know - from getting into school to getting your first job as a nurse and beyond. You will find:

+ Information on the nursing profession and the many career options, including what makes a good nurse and what nursing is *really* like.
+ Help for determining the type of nursing program that's right for you, applying for admission, and finding financial aid.
+ Comprehensive advice and study tips to get you through school, from organization and study skills to minimizing anxiety in exams.
+ The inside scoop on clinicals - what they are like and what you will be expected to do, from care plans to nursing interventions.
+ The lowdown on the NCLEX exam - what it is, how it works and how you can best prepare for it.
+ Tips for balancing school, work and family, making time for yourself and staying motivated through the rough times.
+ Information on grad school and advanced practice nursing specialties.
+ Advice for finding your dream job, writing a resume that gets you noticed, acing employment interviews and evaluating job offers.
+ Insight, inside information and encouragement to help you succeed during your first six months as a practicing professional nurse.

From start to finish, this book has you covered!

So you wanna be a nurse? Don't go at it alone! Use this book as a guide to the career of your dreams. And, use your courage, hard work and determination to make those dreams a reality.

Part I

Before you start out on the road to nursing, you need to
define where you want to go and how you plan to get
there. Getting Started takes a look at the nursing
profession, your career options, and how to select the
right educational path to meet your goals.

The Scoop on Nursing

Before you invest significant time and money into any educational program, it's always a good idea to do a little field homework. Will there be jobs for you after you graduate? What level of education and experience is required for new job seekers? What can you expect, in terms of income and advancement potential? What is the job really like?

We know you want to help people, and perhaps you've dreamed about nursing since you were three. But will it put food on your table? As an occupation, can you depend on it? Absolutely! Nurses are in demand and will continue to be so long into the future.

Why Nursing is Hot

As a career, nursing promises three things: portability, flexibility and ironclad stability. Wherever you go, however your needs change, nursing has a job for you.

The healthcare industry is booming. Industry analysts foresee a 26% increase in jobs through 2008. Nursing is at the forefront, with the most jobs and the most growth:

Fact

+ Registered nursing is the largest healthcare occupation in the US.
+ Currently, there are over 2.2 million jobs for RNs.
+ Out of all occupations, registered nursing ranks in the top ten for greatest projected number of new jobs.

If you are looking for a profession with a promising future, nursing can't be beat.

Why is nursing seeing so much growth? Several factors come in to play. The elderly, who typically have more complex healthcare needs, are seeing a faster than average growth rate in population. Baby boomers are following close behind, bringing with them an alarming rise in heart disease. To top things off, an overwhelming number of experienced nurses are nearing retirement, and as they leave the field, their jobs will need to be filled. The average age of current nursing professionals is now just over 44 years old. Finally, medical advances now allow for the diagnosis and treatment of more conditions and illnesses than ever before thus adding to the demand for qualified nurses.

For the next few years, expect to see pay rates increasing, more attractive benefit packages and flexible work schedules as the industry looks for ways to attract more people to the field.

LPN vs. RN - What's the Difference?

Licensed Practical Nurses (LPNs or LVNs for Licensed Vocational Nurses) and Registered Nurses (RNs) are both considered "nurses," and both are required to pass a national licensing exam after completing an accredited nursing program. The difference between the two is in the scope of practice and responsibilities, as well as the required level of education.

LPNs undergo one year of intensive training in a state-approved program, while RNs must obtain a 2 or 4-year college degree. While both provide basic nursing care, RNs generally have a wider clinical scope of practice and more managerial responsibilities. Additionally, RNs typically have higher earnings and greater opportunity for advancement.

I should also mention that you might come across the term Diploma Nurse. Although most of these instructional programs have vanished, a Diploma Nurse is an RN who has undergone at least 3 years of nursing training. These programs are not degree granting and are normally associated with hospitals and not college or university schools of nursing. Diploma nurses must pass the same state boards as the 2 and 4-year degree RNs.

Which option is best for you will depend on many factors that we'll discuss in the coming chapters, but for now, here are some basic facts to consider:

Fact

+ On average, RNs earn $12,000 a year more than LPNs.
+ Employment options for RNs will be greatest, with more available jobs and more new positions being created.
+ Employment for LPNs in long-term care settings is solid, but they will face stiff competition for hospital jobs.

Let's also take a look at the 2 and 4-year RNs. Does it matter which degree you get? In terms of practice, no. An RN with an associate's degree is licensed to perform the same functions as an RN with a bachelor's degree. In terms of salary, the difference is not really significant - typically a dollar an hour more. So why bother with the bachelor's degree? More flexibility, better opportunities.

Depending on your career goals, the bachelor's degree gives you more options. Four-year RNs complete the same core courses and clinicals as their 2-year counterparts, but they also receive a broad liberal arts education to supplement the nursing program. If you want to go into management, research or advanced practice, the bachelor's degree is the way to go.

More Choices than Stars in the Sky

Gone are the days of ward nursing. Modern nurses enjoy a wide range of career options with enough variety and flexibility to suit every personality. Here's a peek at just some of the specialty areas in which nurses practice:

Ambulatory Care Nursing
Burn Unit Nursing
Cardiac/Cardiovascular Nursing
Case Management
Community Health Nursing
Correctional Nursing
Critical Care Nursing
Emergency Nursing
Flight Nursing
Forensic Nursing
Gastroenterology Nursing
Holistic Nursing
Home Health Nursing
Hospice/Palliative Care
Hyperbaric Nursing
IV Therapy Nursing
Infectious

Disease/Immunology
Lactation Consultant
Legal Nursing
Medical-Surgical Nursing
Metabolic Nursing
Neonatal Nursing
Nephrology Nursing
Neuro-Surgical Nursing
Nurse Anesthetist
Nurse Educator
Nurse Entrepreneur
Nurse Midwife
Nurse Practitioner
Nurse Recruiter
Nursing Informatics
Nursing Management
Obstetrics and Gynecology
Occupational Health Nursing

Oncology Nursing
Ophthalmologic Nursing
Pain Management
Parish Nursing
Pediatric Nursing
Perioperative Nursing
Plastic & Reconstructive Surgery
Psychiatric Nursing
Pulmonary Nursing
Rehabilitation Nursing
Research
School Nursing
Sports Medicine Nursing
Telephone Triage Nursing
Transplant Nursing
Travel Nursing
Urology Nursing
Wound Care

The range of roles available to nurses allows for unique job opportunities that are compatible with and complement outside interests:

+ Need "mother's hours," so you can be home when your children are? Try School Nursing.
+ Looking for the variety and excitement of the jet-set life? See the world with Travel Nursing.
+ Like detective work? Forensic Nursing is right up your alley.
+ Interested in law? Legal nursing might be just for you.
+ Wanting to try virus hunting, as seen in *Hot Zone* or *Outbreak?* Join the ranks of immunology and infectious disease nurses.
+ Got sports fever? There are nurse specialists in Sports Medicine, too!

You will be exposed to many of these areas during clinicals, where you will have the opportunity to learn first-hand which areas of practice you enjoy. For now, rest assured that there are enough career options to meet your goals and then some. The possibilities are endless - the choices are up to you!

Chapter 2

Is Nursing For You?

How do you know if nursing will be a good fit for you? The first step is to check your motivation - why do you want to be a nurse?

Watch Out

Many people who felt "called" to nursing have been disappointed by its reality. Romantic visions of "ER" heroism or saintly bedside vigils are rarely borne out. Nursing has more than its share of touching moments and rewarding experiences, but make no mistake: it is HARD work, and rarely glamorous. If your motivation is to feel needed, nursing is not for you. If you need external praise or gratitude to feel good about yourself and your work, again, nursing is not for you.

Another myth has it that becoming a nurse is easier than pursuing other healthcare occupations. Nothing could be further from the truth. Nursing programs are extremely difficult, at best - heavy on the science and math courses, brutally time-intensive and physically draining. It takes serious commitment and a strong sense of self to succeed in nursing school. For some, nursing school is the single greatest challenge of their lives. If you are looking for an easy degree, nursing is not for you.

Also consider that your nursing degree is not the end of the line - in truth, it is just the beginning of your education. The medical world evolves and changes rapidly. New advances in technology and treatment, the emergence of new diseases and conditions, and the shifting needs of an aging population make it critical for nurses to keep abreast of developments in the healthcare field. Enormous quantities of information come out each year - you have to be able to keep up with it. Continuing education is a requirement of nursing, so if you are put off at the thought of "life-long learning," nursing is not for you.

What, then, are the right reasons for going into nursing? You will need to ask that question of yourself, as only you can determine the right answer; but know this: if your motivation is internal and sincere, you are on the right track.

Why Nursing?

I want to feel like what I do matters. I want to touch people's lives, to soothe their pains, to comfort them in their losses, to share their joys, to help them heal. I want to leave my job at the end of the day knowing that what I did during my shift mattered, that I filled a need for someone that day. I can think of no career more noble, and no cause more worthy - I want to be a part of that.

- Louise Komorek, BSN student
Southern Illinois University

Student Nurse Snapshot

What is the typical nursing student like? The answers may surprise you. According to the Health Resources and Services Administration, Division of Nursing, the average age of new nursing students is now 29 years old, up from 23 in 1977. Nursing attracts a large proportion of non-traditional students as well - returning adult students pursuing a second career, and professionals maintaining outside employment while in school. Many nursing students have families to care for, which places additional demands on their time. A major challenge for today's nursing student is finding a reasonable way to balance family, work and school.

Nursing remains a primarily female profession, but the number of male nurses is on the rise, currently at 9%. Minorities are also under represented at 10% of the nursing population, but are experiencing the fastest growth rate of all new professionals as the field of nursing continues its efforts to diversify.

Close to two thirds of the nation's nursing students are enrolled in LPN programs or associate's degree programs, the remainder pursuing a bachelor's degree at the outset. There is also a separate population of currently licensed professionals who have elected to return to school. These students have chosen to complete their degree through fast-track programs (more commonly called "bridge" programs). This group of students includes LPNs bridging to RN, and 2-year RNs bridging to the bachelor's or master's degree.

What Makes A Good Nurse?

Until he extends his circle of compassion to include all living things, man will not himself find peace.

- Albert Schweitzer

What makes a good nurse? There isn't a set criteria or magic formula - the best nurses draw on their own unique strengths, bringing diversity to the profession. In general, though, there are certain qualities that all great nurses share:

> ✦ **Empathy** - the ability to connect with others through compassion and understanding.
> ✦ **Tolerance** - respect for diversity and the capacity for non-judgmental, objective delivery of care; able to recognize the intrinsic value of every human being.
> ✦ **Strong organizational skills** - capable of prioritizing, managing a large workload and carrying out tasks efficiently; adept at time management and highly organized.

✦ **Well-developed critical thinking skills** - able to use good judgement and act responsibly under stressful conditions; strong problem solving abilities and a high level of initiative.

✦ **Excellent communication skills** - able to relate complex concepts in an manner more easily understood; solid social and interpersonal skills; capable of developing positive relationships with patients, peers and superiors.

Many capable nurses have flawless technique and a formidable knowledge base, but the truly exceptional nurse offers something more. Great nurses are positive thinkers, mentors, leaders and supporters. They are advocates, educators and scientists. Above all, they are healers - of body, mind and spirit.

A Day in the Life

There is no "typical" day for nurses - ask any one of them and they will tell you to expect the unexpected! In general though, you will:

✦ develop and implement care plans.

✦ monitor and assess the condition of your patients.

✦ provide bedside care.

✦ take vital signs, collect samples and perform routine lab tests.

✦ administer medications, injections or other treatment; and

✦ care for wounds and incisions.

Additionally, you may instruct patients in self-care, assist with surgical procedures, provide emergency interventions, assist with patient hygiene, counsel family members and supervise aides. If you are an RN, you might also start IV therapies, blood transfusions, and perform other advanced clinical procedures.

As a nurse, you will participate in a team-oriented environment composed of many healthcare professionals, technicians and administrative staff. In most settings, you will be the main provider of hands-on care. Physicians and techs may only be able to spend a few minutes a day with patients, while nurses interact with all their patients throughout each shift. The team will rely on you to monitor and advocate for your patients' needs.

But What is it Really Like?

No matter what field you work in, there will always be office politics, burnt-out employees and gossipmongers. Put together a diverse group of people who must depend on each other in stressful situations, and conflicts are bound to arise. But what of drawbacks specific to nursing?

Watch Out

There are some negatives that come with the territory. As licensed healthcare professionals, nurses are legally accountable for their practice. The title comes with serious responsibilities, which, when not adhered to, have equally serious consequences. That's just the nature of the game. Laws are in place to protect the consumers, and rightfully so. You need to be aware that if you are negligent or provide substandard care, you could be held professionally, and in some instances personally, liable.

Nursing can also be a high-stress job, depending on your area of practice. Long hours, sicker patients and understaffing in some facilities puts a lot of pressure on the nursing staff. Shift work is the rule, not the exception, and day shift openings are hard to come by for new graduates.

Finally, nursing is not just taking care of people...nursing also involves paperwork - LOTS of paperwork. Charting and other forms of documentation can take up almost as much time as caring for your patients.

So what's the trade-off? You will never be bored, you will never have any two days alike, and the work is always interesting. Everyday will bring with it the chance to learn something new and to make a real difference in the lives of others...that's what it's all about. If you want a truly rewarding, satisfying career, nursing is the one.

Testing the Waters Before Diving in

One of the best things you can do before applying to nursing school is to work in the field. For example, working as a Certified Nurse Aide (CNA) or medical technician will give you valuable insight into the healthcare field, and will allow you to evaluate nursing. It's important for you to know if nursing is right for you.

Working in the field will:

Tip

- ✦ Allow you to perfect basic patient care skills, so you can focus more fully on learning nursing techniques in clinicals.
- ✦ Familiarize you with medical terminology, acronyms, common medications/conditions and nursing lingo.
- ✦ Expose you to the hospital or long term care environment, helping you to understand clinical protocols.
- ✦ Introduce you to experienced LPNs and RNs - potential mentors from whom you can learn and ask for guidance.
- ✦ Demonstrate your commitment to the field when you apply to nursing school. It looks great on your application, especially when followed up with a letter of reference from your employer.

And finally, getting your feet wet first could come in handy down the line when you are looking for your first nursing job.

Ask

Most community colleges offer 6 to 8 week CNA training programs that are fairly cost-effective (usually less than the cost of a 3-credit hour college course). After you have completed training, you can take the certification exam. For more information, call your local community college and ask about their allied health training programs.

If you do not have the time or flexibility to work as a CNA, another way to gain quality experience is through volunteer work. Hospitals, clinics and long term care facilities are always looking for volunteers, and are willing to work within your schedule. By offering to help out, you are providing a valuable community service while gaining first-hand exposure to the healthcare field.

Chapter 3

First Things First

Now is the time to think long and hard about what you want to accomplish in your nursing career, and which path you need to follow to get there. You will need to decide what level of licensure and education you want. You will then need to find the right program to meet those goals. Finally, you need to work on developing a stellar nursing school application - one that makes you stand out in the selective admissions process.

Planning Your Path

*"If you can find a path with no obstacles,
it probably doesn't go anywhere."*

- Anonymous

The choice about what kind of nursing education to pursue is a highly personal one. There is no "best" way to go, other than what works for your own situation.

You may have already heard some grumbling about which is the better nurse - the LPN, the 2-year RN or the 4-year RN. Let it go in one ear and out the other. The truth is both LPNs and RNs (2 or 4 year) are highly skilled, trained nurses. Both are equally deserving of respect and admiration for their hard work, clinical expertise and compassionate care. When deciding whether to be an LPN or an RN, you need to determine what will be best for YOU.

Set aside some time to reflect on the following issues:
+ **Time Commitment** - How much time are you able to devote to schooling? 1 year? 4 years? Bear in mind that most nursing programs are set up to run Monday through Friday, full-time, days. It is rare to find programs with night or weekend learning options. This will limit your ability to work while in school and may affect your financial situation.
+ **Finances** - There is plenty of help available through grants and scholarships to offset the cost of school itself, but you need to think about living expenses. Will you need to work while in school? Are there ways you can cut down on your household expenses? If student loans are needed to help you get by, how much debt you are willing to take on? When you are budgeting, take into consideration the added cost of textbooks (you will own a library by the time you are through with school), testing fees, extended daycare for when clinicals run late, gas for travelling to distant clinical assignments, liability insurance, tools of the trade (uniforms, stethoscope, etc.), and so on.
+ **Work** - If you will be working your way through school, how flexible is your employer? Are you able to cut back to part-time work? During clinical rotations, you will typically be in school from 7:00 a.m. to 5:00 p.m. You will also need time to study, read, write care plans and complete homework - an additional three hours per day minimum.

- ◆ **Family** - Do you have a spouse? Children? What kinds of family responsibilities do you have? There are many ways to balance school and family, the best of which is to encourage their support by getting them involved. Are family members willing to help out more with household chores? Do you have back-up daycare providers? What plan of action can you implement if one of your children gets sick, or if school is cancelled for a snow day?
- ◆ **Prior Education** - Do you have any previous college experience? Most nursing programs have prerequisite courses - classes you need to complete before starting their program. This could add an extra year to your education - something to keep in mind when planning finances.
- ◆ **Prior Experience** - Have you worked as a CNA or volunteered at a healthcare facility? Any exposure to the field at all? While not always required, admissions committees *really* like to see this on an application.
- ◆ **Career Goals** - What is your destination? Are you planning to go into advanced practice, specialization or management? Which works best for your situation - getting the 4-year degree up-front, or completing the 2-year degree, working for a few years, then bridging to the bachelor's?

Remember, choosing which nursing path to pursue is a personal decision - you need to evaluate what will be best for your own lifestyle, needs and goals. Keep the above issues in mind as you prepare for nursing school. Going in with your eyes open will help smooth out some of the bumps in the road along the way.

Selecting a Program

When evaluating nursing programs, the first thing to check is accreditation. Your nursing program needs to be accredited by the *National League of Nursing's Accreditation Committee* or by the *Commission on Collegiate Nursing Education*. It should also be "approved" by your state's Board of Nursing or Department of Education. If your program is approved but not accredited, your license may not transfer to other states - something to keep in mind. It's best to find an accredited program to keep your options open.

More than likely, there will be several accredited programs in your area. Factors to consider when narrowing down your choices include cost, distance, entrance requirements and program structure. Request an information packet from local schools for the basics on the program, then follow up with a personal tour. Most nursing programs host an open house in the fall and spring, where you will have the opportunity to ask questions and see the facilities.

Tip

If possible, talk with current nursing students - how do they like the program? Do they feel they are getting a good education? Are they happy with their choice? Why or why not?

When all is said and done, one or two nursing programs will stand out as most closely matching your criteria; however it's a good idea to apply to several programs - this will give you more options when the time comes to make your final decision.

A Word on Distance Learning

Distance learning is becoming an extremely popular educational alternative for working professionals and other non-traditional students whose schedules or family responsibilities prevent them from physically attending class. Most colleges now offer select classes (and in some cases, complete degree programs) over the internet. Using chat rooms, message boards, web sites, e-mail and other technology based tools to communicate, instructors are able to deliver course material and advise students throughout the term.

Unfortunately, due to the unique nature of nursing, there are very few distance learning options for entry-level programs at this time, although there are many options for nurses who are already licensed. This is, in part, because supervised clinical experience is critical to the learning process.

Excelsior College (formerly *Regents*) is one of the few accredited nursing programs available for distance learners. Their RN programs are designed specifically for working professionals with *significant* experience in clinically-oriented healthcare disciplines (such as EMTs, paramedics, LPNs, respiratory therapists, etc.). You can earn your associate's or bachelor's degree through Excelsior, but you will need to provide documented proof of prior clinical experience to be considered for admission. Entrance requirements are very strict in this regard.

Watch Out

Also note that *some* states do not license Regents grads - check first to make sure the degree is approved in your state. Be aware that Excelsior's program is very challenging and quite costly.

Ask

For more information, contact:
Excelsior College
7 Columbia Circle
Albany, NY 12203-5159
1-888-647-2388

For those nurses who are currently licensed RNs, there are *many* options for degree completion or advanced studies. Most colleges now offer distance learning programs for bridging (RN to BSN) and master's degrees.

Entrance Exams

Not all schools have them, but nursing entrance exams are a fairly popular tool used by colleges to assist in the student selection and placement process. The intent of the entrance exams is NOT to test you on your knowledge of nursing or the medical field; rather, they test for basic math, science and verbal skills.

Common tests include the *RNEE (Registered Nurse Entrance Exam)*, *PNEE (Practical Nurse Entrance Exam)*, *HOBET (Health Occupations Basic Entrance Test)*, *NET (Nurse Entrance Test)*, and the *NPEE (Nursing Pre-Entrance Exam)*. Additionally, international students will need to take the *TOEFL (Test of English as a Foreign Language)*.

Don't Panic

Should you stress out about entrance exams? No. While many schools do have a minimum score you need to achieve, the tests are not that bad - honest! Still, if you have been out of school for a long period of time, or if you feel nervous, there are several exam prep books you can purchase at your local bookstore, or check out of the library. Preparing ahead of time with exam prep resources can help build your confidence. The main thing here is to go into the test with a positive attitude.

Pre-Flight Checklist

OK, you know where you want to go, and what type of nurse you want to be - you are almost ready! Here's a final list of the things you will need to complete before applying to nursing school:

❑ **Take the ACTs, SATs and any other required college entrance exams**
   Most often, the ACT and SAT are taken in high school and will carry over; however, some programs do require that the tests be taken within the preceding three years. If this is the case, you may need to take them again - ask about your school's policy. Also, find out which, if any, nursing entrance exams are required. LPN programs may require CNA certification prior to admission.

❑ **Complete prerequisite courses**
   Contact the school you are applying to for a list of prerequisites. If you are attending community college and plan to transfer into a 4-year university for the nursing program, make sure your courses transfer. While you are not required to have all prerequisites completed at the time you apply, you will need to have them done before the nursing program starts.

❑ **Get letters of recommendation**

You may be asked to furnish several letters of recommendation with your application. Typically, admissions committees will want to see recommendations from a previous employer (preferably in the healthcare field), a college professor and a third person of your choosing who can provide a character reference. This could be your church pastor or priest, a volunteer coordinator you have worked with, or a member of any professional organizations to which you belong. Try to stay away from using family and friends as references.

The Application Process

All nursing programs have what is called a "selective admissions policy." This means you are not automatically guaranteed a spot, even if you meet all the initial admissions requirements. You will be competing with many other students for a limited number of open spots (note that it is not unusual for a college to attract 3 to 5 times more applicants than they have room for). Additionally, most programs only start once a year. If you don't make it in the first time, you may have a year's wait on your hands before you will be able to try again.

Because of this, it is critical that you have your ducks in a row:

Don't Forget

♦ Make sure you meet ALL admissions requirements. This includes having your prerequisites complete or near completion, and meeting the stated minimum grade point average (GPA).

♦ Turn in a *complete* application. Make sure everything has been filled out, signed, and is accompanied by all requested documentation (letters of recommendation, application fee, essay, transcripts to school, test scores, etc.)

♦ Get the application in AS EARLY AS POSSIBLE.

How can you make your application stand out among hundreds of other qualified students? What are admissions committees looking for?

What Makes An Applicant Stand Out?

◆ Excellent grades, especially in science courses (anatomy, physiology, microbiology and chemistry)

◆ Health-related experiences, whether paid, volunteer or both (ideally)

◆ General volunteer experiences - are you a good *community* citizen?

◆ Leadership experiences

◆ Strong, supportive letters of recommendation

What Are the Top Three MOST Important Factors?

◆ Grades - You must be a strong student to succeed in this rigorous academic program and profession

◆ Nursing-related experiences - What have you done to foster your interest in the nursing profession?

◆ Strong letters of recommendation - Ask the people you feel you know best and will speak highly of you as a potential nurse. A less-than-stellar letter of recommendation can be damaging to your chances of getting into your preferred school of nursing.

- Cynthia Schudel, Admissions Advisor/Recruiter
University of Kansas School of Nursing

Writing a Powerful Entrance Essay

Tip

Along with your application, you may be asked to write an essay - typically on why you want to be a nurse. Please, *please* do not write, "Because I want to help people." Everyone who wants to be a nurse is interested in helping people - the committee knows that already and your essay will blend right in with all the other applications. "If you just want to help people," they will say, "there are hundreds of other professions you can go into." Ah...so the question *really* reads, "Why do you want to be a NURSE?"

They are looking for two things: what will nursing do for you and what will you do for nursing? Put yourself in the shoes of the admissions committee, who must decide which students to accept. As they review each application and essay, they will be asking:

◆ How much thought have you put into this? Have you sat down and developed goals for your future career? Showing the admissions committee you have a plan for your career lets them know you are committed.

◆ What are you going to do to develop, enhance or otherwise further the profession? What are you going to give back to the nursing community? Do you have a dedicated vision? Remember, their goal is not just to churn out new graduates. Their goal is to mentor and develop the future leaders of the field.

The essay is your chance to express why nursing is the field for you and what you hope to accomplish as a nurse. It's your best opportunity to showcase your strengths and convey a bit of your personality. Keep these things in mind, take your time with it, and write with sincerity. Double check your spelling and grammar, and have at least one other person read it and review it for you. Your efforts will pay off in the form of a great essay!

The Interview

Once you have submitted your application, all required documentation and your essay, you may be called in for an interview with a member of the committee. Don't panic. Think of it as your chance to shine.

Remember that recurring Saturday Night Live skit, *Daily Affirmations with Stuart Smalley?* "I'm good enough, I'm smart enough, and gosh darn it, people like me!" Well, you ARE good enough - you always have been, and now is no time to be someone else. Just be yourself. They want to get to know you better.

Here is some more advice on the interview:

> **Be Prepared**
> If attending a face-to-face interview, be prepared:
> ✦ Have extra copies of your essay, resume and transcripts.
> ✦ Look neat and professional
> ✦ Ask questions about the nursing program - do your homework about the program and school.
> ✦ Be concise and thorough, but not repetitious.
> ✦ Identify what exactly is being asked and speak directly to that (don't ramble).
> ✦ Be honest. Don't exaggerate, but don't be afraid to speak about your accomplishments.
>
> - Cynthia Schudel, Advisor/Admissions Counselor
> University of Kansas School of Nursing

Tip

One more bit of advice - you can stress yourself out preparing perfectly scripted answers to the "why do you want to be a nurse" question, but in truth, they may not even ask you that. Go figure! It's better to get plenty of rest the night before, pamper yourself in the morning and go in with a winning positive attitude. Smiling is infectious...and so is sincerity.

Waiting...and Waiting...

You turned in your application months ago. It was the most perfect, complete, stellar application in the history of nursing students. Your interview was fantastic - so great, you were sure they would offer you a spot right then and there. And yet...the mailbox is oddly empty. The cobwebs are starting to collect cobwebs, and - was that just a tumbleweed blowing past?

Rest easy...it takes forever to get that acceptance letter. Entire seasons pass. Really. Most colleges don't send out acceptance letters until the spring...so if you applied in September, don't panic when you have not received word by January. The letter will come sometime in March or April.

Keeping Your Piggy Bank Happy

Unless you happen to be independently wealthy, the cost of attending nursing school is a big concern. You may have children and a household to support. You may be a first-time college student without financial resources. Tuition, fees, books, living expenses - where is it all going to come from? Let's look at your options, starting off with employment.

Work and School - Can it Be Done?

Is it realistic for you to work full-time while in school? There *are* students who have successfully managed nursing school while working full-time in the evenings and on weekends, but this is extremely rare. The time commitment required of nursing students is greater than that of the average college student. The schedule is less flexible. Homework and studying are more time-intensive, and don't forget clinicals. Realistically, full-time employment and nursing school are not compatible for the majority of students. That's the bad news. The good news is you may not need to work full-time.

When it comes to paying for college, there is help to be had - and plenty of it. There is an incredible amount of financial assistance available to you, if you are willing to spend a little time researching your options.

Paying for College: Myths vs. Reality

If money doesn't grow on trees,
how come banks have so many branches?

- Anonymous

Think you can't afford college? Think again! Did you know a total of 64 billion dollars in aid is available to help students in the U.S., through grants, scholarships and low-interest loans? Or that one in five traditional-aged undergraduate students come from families whose annual income is less than $20,000 a year? Help is out there - all you need to do is ask. Here are some more myths we can dispel:

Myth #1: College costs $100,000 a year.
Okay, obviously this is not true - but it sure seems like it, doesn't it? Actually, you'd be surprised - college is not really out of your reach. You can attend a community college for as little as $1,700 a year, and some state universities for around $3,500 a year. At the other end of the spectrum a private university will run you about $12,000 per year for full-time studies, but this cost is frequently offset by financial aid.

Myth #2: Even at "only" a couple thousand a year, I can't afford it.
What? You mean you don't have a spare $12,000 collecting dust in your cookie jar? Take heart - you are not the only one. In fact, most people don't have that kind of cash flow available. But you don't have to bear the entire cost of college on your own. There are grants, scholarships, loans, employer-sponsored tuition reimbursement plans, and tuition-for-service programs available to help you out.

Myth #3: You have to be a straight-A student or star athlete to qualify for scholarships.
This is the biggest myth, by far. The fact is most scholarships and grants are awarded based on *financial need*. Seven out of 10 full-time undergraduate students receive financial aid. More than half of all students receive government grants, and the average annual award is just under $4,000.

Grants and Scholarships

By far, the best kind of aid to get is grants and scholarships. These funds can be applied to tuition, books, fees, and in some cases, living expenses. Grants and scholarships do not have to be repaid.

The majority of grants come from the federal government. The most common award is the Pell Grant, which is based solely on financial need. For many, the Pell Grant is a foundation to which other forms of aid can be added. When you visit your college's financial aid office, you will be asked to fill out a form called the FASFA (Free Application for Federal Student Aid). The college uses this to generate an SAR (Student Aid Report), so they can find as much assistance for you as possible. You are automatically considered for a Pell Grant when you fill out this form.

Scholarships are available at the local, state and national level. There are scholarships specifically for nursing students, scholarships you may qualify for based on affiliation (such as those offered by employers and the armed forces) and scholarships awarded for academic excellence. These are not automatically applied for with the FASFA, but your financial aid advisor will help you investigate your options.

Watch Out

Beware of companies that offer to find you scholarships for a fee. Your college financial aid office will help you find all the aid you need - *free of charge*.

For more information on government-sponsored assistance, write to:
Federal Student Aid Information Center
P.O. Box 84
Washington, D.C. 20044-0084
1-800-4-FED-AID

Student Loans

The government offers loans to help students pay for the remaining costs of college after grants and scholarships. The most common loan is the Stafford Loan. The Stafford Loan is available to undergraduate students attending college at least part-time. Subsidized loans (interest-free) are awarded based on financial need. Unsubsidized loans are not need-based, and interest is added to the principal.

Generally, you can borrow up to $5500 a year in subsidized loans, and another $5,000 in unsubsidized loans. The money must first be applied to tuition, books, fees and, if you live on campus, room and board. Any remaining funds can be used for living expenses.

Ask

You do not start paying on your loan until 6 months after you graduate, leave school or drop down to less than part-time enrollment. This grace period gives you time to find a job and get settled. For more information on federal loans, call 1-800-4-FED-AID.

There are other non-government loans available, as well. Your financial aid advisor will help you investigate your options if more help is needed.

Still More Types of Aid

Didn't we promise there was plenty of help available to make college affordable? In addition to grants, scholarships and loans, there are a few more options to help you pay for school:

✦ **Employer-Sponsored Tuition Reimbursement** - Many health care employers offer tuition reimbursement as a benefit. You pay the cost of school up front, and at the end of each semester, if you have satisfactory grades, they reimburse your expenses. Check with your Human Resources Department to see if your employer offers this type of program.

✦ **Tuition-For Service Loan Repayment Programs** - Many of the larger healthcare corporations will offer to repay part of your student loans in exchange for an agreement to work for them for a set period of time. Again, consult the Human Resources Department. The federal government offers a similar repayment program if you are willing to work in rural or under-served areas where there is a nursing shortage. In exchange for a contractual agreement to work 2 years in an approved facility, they will repay up to 60% of your school loans. For more information on the federal program, contact:

bandidobooks.com

Nursing Education Loan Repayment Program
Loan Repayment Programs Branch
Division of Scholarships and Loan Repayments
Bureau of Primary Health Center
4350 East-West Highway, 10th Floor
Bethesda, MD 20814
1-800-435-6464

Part II

Once you are in nursing school, the real work begins. This section will walk you step by step from your first day in class to the day you graduate. All the tools you need are included, giving you a master blueprint for success!

Gearing Up for Student Life

Congratulations - you've made it! You are now an official nursing student. Expect to be both excited and terrified for the next few months as you eagerly await your first day in class.

Don't Panic

The natural impulse is to start reading everything you can get your hands on about nursing to prepare for school. It seems logical - and let's face it - you can't *wait* to be a nurse. You want to know everything *now*. As hard as it may be, resist this urge with all your might. Why? There are several reasons:

+ The summer before your nursing program starts is the LAST free time you will have until you graduate. Nursing school runs year-round; it's better to take advantage of the precious time you have left to tend to all things non-nursing in nature.
+ You risk an early burnout. Nursing programs are unlike anything you have experienced, and really, it's best to save your energy for the program.
+ You deserve to take time to reward yourself. You've worked hard to get into nursing school - don't shrug it off. It's important for you to recognize what a tremendous accomplishment this is.

Take some time now to celebrate, pamper yourself and relax for a while. The next opportunity to do this will be years down the road. Spend some quality time with your friends and family, get outside, and have some fun!

"But there must be *something* we can work on now - isn't there?" you plead, "Formulas we should memorize or diseases we should read up on? Anything?" Alright, if you insist on having something nursing-related to do over the summer...try boning up on medical terminology or medical prefixes and suffixes. Granted, its not as exciting as, say, learning to read an EKG or studying the latest nursing theories, but it will serve you well in your schooling and save you endless headaches later on.

One thing you *will* need to take care of the summer before you begin nursing school is the pre-entrance checklist. Your nursing program will require documentation of the following before the first day of class:

+ **Physical Exam**
  You will be required to have a physical exam. Your nursing program will provide a form for your health care provider to fill out stating that you are physically able to participate in the program.
+ **Immunizations**
  While you are getting your physical, you will also need to get documentation proving your immunizations are up-to-date. If your records are not available, a simple blood test can be done to measure antibody titers in your system. This test will show what boosters you need. Also note that you made need certain tests to participate in clinicals, such as tuberculosis and hepatitis screens.

✦ **Dental Exam**

This one is not required by all programs, but I have heard of some that do require a visit to the dentist before school starts. If this is required, you will get the dental form and information in your orientation packet.

✦ **CPR certification**

Proof of current certification in cardiopulmonary resuscitation (CPR) is almost always required prior to beginning nursing school and you will be required to keep your certification active throughout the program. While some programs are setup to offer the course as part of the curriculum, check with your nursing program ahead of time to see what the requirements are. While you are on the phone with them, ask what kind of certification is required -"basic CPR" or "CPR for healthcare professionals." The American Red Cross offers affordable courses in CPR that meet this requirement. Call your local affiliate for course offerings in your area.

✦ **Insurance**

You will be required to have valid health insurance prior to the program start, and may need malpractice/liability insurance for clinicals. Your school will be able to direct you to low-cost student insurance options if you do not have your own.

Tools of the Trade

Now we're getting to the fun stuff. Not just school supplies, but *nursing* supplies. Oooooh...ahhhhhh... Sends little shivers of excitement down your spine, doesn't it?

There are some tools of the trade you will need to purchase for nursing school. While required items for each program vary, the following equipment is fairly typical:

✦ Nursing uniform or scrubs.
✦ Nursing shoes.
✦ Wristwatch with a second hand.
✦ Stethoscope.
✦ Bandage scissors.
✦ Pen light.

Other items you may need include a lab coat, goggles, a blood pressure cuff, a CPR mask with non-returnable vent and a reflex hammer. Consult your program for a specific list of required items.

Tip

Before you go rushing off to the nearest medical supply store to drop $500 on state-of-the-art gear, let's look at the quality requirements. For most of the above items, generic will do. Save your money on those so you can invest in the items where quality *does* matter, specifically nursing shoes and a stethoscope.

It pays to invest in a higher-end nursing shoe, trust me. When you are looking at long hours on your feet, good nursing shoes can spare you back and foot problems down the road. Make sure they fit well, provide ample support and are comfortable. For male students, white sneakers are a comparable alternative to the traditional nursing shoe. Also note that while unisex nursing clogs have become popular in recent years, you should check for specific uniform restrictions before purchasing a pair - some programs do not allow them.

As for a stethoscope, those in the medium price range will serve you well. You don't need the $200 cardiology stethoscope for nursing school, but then again, the $10 models are going to be harder to hear through. Pick something in the middle that you like. Nursing uniforms vary from program to program, so you may not have much flexibility on the style or vendor. Just know that you will need more than one. Some students even buy 5 uniforms to save on laundry time during the week, but 3 should be sufficient.

Meet Your New Family

> *We are not primarily put on this earth to see through one another,*
> *but to see one another through.*
>
> Peter de Vries

Your fellow classmates - you will eat with them, study with them, laugh with them and cry with them. You will live and breathe nursing with them. For the next few years, these folks will be the only people who understand and empathize with what you are going through.

You need to know how important your relationship with your classmates will be to succeeding in nursing school. Up until now, school has probably been a solo act. Sure, you've made friends in your prerequisite classes, but primarily you have been responsible for you alone, and it has worked well. Nothing could be further from the truth in nursing school.

Nursing school is a team effort that requires mutual cooperation, respect and care. It is only by working together that you can succeed. As a group, you will depend on each other for support, collegial sharing, motivation and courage. By the time you get through nursing school, your classmates will know more about you (and vice versa) than some of your best friends and family members.

The **Special Rule of Nursing Relativity** guarantees that:

+ The student you don't get along with will be the one you have to practice injections on.
+ The student who knows-it-all will be the one who must do a complete physical exam on you; and
+ The student so flighty she has her own orbit will be the one assigned to work clinicals with you.

Fortunately, the **Special Rule of Nursing Relativity** also guarantees that:

+ The student who initially seemed so unfriendly will be the one to surprise you with help before a test.
+ The student you blew off will be the one who offers you comfort after a rough clinical experience; and
+ The student you found most eccentric will grow to become one of your closest friends and staunchest allies.

Take care when developing relationships with your classmates. Don't fall into the gossip trap and above all, suspend judgement. Every person in nursing school has earned the right to be there and brings unique personal qualities to the table. Learn from each other and grow together.

Student Survival Skills 101

What's the number one predictor of success in class? Studying faithfully every night?
Nope. Taping lectures and dutifully transcribing them after each class? Nope.
Highlighting notes and textbooks in 10 different colors? Nope, wrong again. The
number one predictor of success in class is (drum roll please...):

Attendance

Could it be that merely showing up for school is the single best thing you can do to
succeed? Absolutely! Go to class every single day. It's that simple. Even the best
students suffer when they miss classes, and struggling students improve their grades by
leaps and bounds simply by showing up for all the lectures.

Ask

Additionally, most nursing programs have *very strict* attendance policies - especially
when it comes to clinicals. Make sure that you are familiar with all of your program's
rules and regulations, especially the attendance policy.

With this in mind, let's look at some of the other equally painless tips and tricks students use to succeed in nursing school. These basic survival skills employ an easy-to-
use, common-sense approach to student life and learning that will make a tremendous
difference for you in school.

Getting Organized

*We are what we repeatedly do. Excellence is therefore
not an act, but a habit.*

- Aristotle

Staying organized is without a doubt one of *the* most important things you can do to
succeed in school. This doesn't mean scheduling every minute of the day or trying to
maintain a sophisticated alpha-numeric file system. For most of us, such things are
unrealistic. Getting organized simply means developing a consistent method to
categorize and store information. Effective systems should require minimal maintenance while allowing you quick access to the information you need. Most importantly,
an effective organizational system should work FOR you.   If it is too cumbersome or
time-consuming, you will not keep it up.

Why bother with organization? It will save you time, allow you to work more
effectively and will help you keep your sanity. Plus, there is a certain positive attitude
boost one gets from feeling on top of things.

Tip

The three basic rules of effective organization are:

+ **Keep it simple.**
  When designing a personal system, simpler is better. The more complicated your system, the less likely you will maintain it.
+ **Keep it central.**
  Keep all your supplies, texts, folders, binders and notebooks in one place. Take only what you need for class each day, and return everything to its designated spot each night.
+ **Keep it current.**
  It's okay to stuff your notes and handouts willy-nilly in your backpack while at school, but once you get home, put them in their place. Faithfully. Every night.

Each student has their own system - you need to find out what works for you. Some students like to arrange all their notes and handouts in one large binder, divided by class. Others like to have a separate folder and notebook for each class. Here are some easy ideas to get you started:

+ **Code it**
  Color-code notebooks, files and folders for each course (i.e. green for Biology, red for Anatomy, etc.). This will make it easier to grab the right materials in a rush.
+ **File it**
  Create a file folder for each course. After every unit exam, place all notes, handouts, returned assignments, quizzes and tests in this folder. This way, everything you need will be handy for midterms and finals.
+ **Date it**
  Put the date and corresponding chapter on all your notes, handouts and tapes. This helps keep things in order, and finding information later will be a breeze.

Another big part of being organized is scheduling your time. Spending just one hour at the beginning of each semester will make your life much less stressful down the road. Purchase a good daily planner. After your first day of classes, sit down in a quiet spot and pull out all your course syllabi.

Tip

Go through your planner and block out your classes for each day of the week (start/end times, classroom, etc.). Using your course outlines, fill in major exam dates/times and note when finals are for each class. Sometimes, there won't be a particular date for a unit exam, but you can usually narrow it down to a specific week. Be sure to also note other important dates you come across (research paper due dates, school holidays, etc.).

Divide up required reading for each class - it will be more manageable and less overwhelming if you break it down into smaller chunks. If you will be covering chapters 1 through 6 in Anatomy during the first three weeks of class, "assign" yourself 2 chapters per week to read. You may want to designate Saturday or Sunday as "reading day" so you will be prepared for each week's lecture.

Maintain your planner by writing in assignments as they come up. Refer to it each night after class, so you will know where things stand. A quick visual overview will help you better prioritize your studies and plan your work. But remember, it doesn't work if you don't use it!

Sharpen Your Study Skills

How many times have you read a couple pages of text, only to discover you have no idea what you just read? Or equally frustrating, you have no idea what parts of it are important? Sometimes, it ALL seems important...but you can't very well memorize an entire text or highlight the entire book.

The keys to good studying are effectiveness, efficiency and consistency. Studying *smarter* is the ultimate goal, which will increase your retention and decrease your stress level.

<u>Tops 10 Tips For Studying Smarter:</u>
1. Same place, same time.
Get into the study habit by designating one area for studying only. Develop a habitual "study period" and stick to it.
2. Get it together.
Gather everything you will need (books, notes, handouts) <u>before</u> you sit down to study.
3. Browse the headlines.
Skim the pages of text you are studying, reading subject headings and bulleted or bold-face information. This is the big picture.
4. Find the moral of the story.
After reading the headlines, ask yourself, "What's important here?" Keep the main ideas and concepts in mind as you go on to study.
5. Have a cup o' joe and read.
Prop your feet up and read the material - don't try to memorize right now...just read it.
6. Snap a picture.
Recap the information in your mind: "Today I learned that there are three types of blood vessels in the body. They are..." Condense and summarize in your own words.
7. Map it out.
Take a few moments to outline the main points and subtopics. Use a method that works for you - write it out or highlight important text.

8. Stack the deck.
Make yourself flashcards for specific information. Put questions on one side of an index card and answers on the other. Include useful definitions, facts and steps (i.e. The steps of DNA replication are...).

9. Play Nursing School Trivia.
Quiz yourself periodically - set aside 30 minutes a night for flashcard quizzes and keep some handy for downtime between classes.

10. Share your toys.
Share your information with your study group. Teaching them helps reinforce the material for you.

Also, DO remember to take breaks. You shouldn't spend more than one hour at a time on any given subject without a break. Get up, walk around, stretch, change the laundry. Give yourself a few minutes to recharge.

See? That's not so bad. Slow and steady wins the race, remember? Consistency in your study habits is the key.

Don't Panic

A final note -you may find in short order that everything I have suggested falls to the wayside. This is normal. I am giving you the tools to start out with good study habits, but the reality of nursing school is that you will *not* have enough time to do everything. Even the most organized, consistent students will find themselves getting up at 4:00 in the morning to study for an exam at 7:00 a.m. You may be looking at 5-6 exams per week, plus homework, *plus* clinicals! You will have to find a system that fits your personal style. Use what you can from the tips I have shared, but adapt things to work for *you*.

Procrastination: The 8th Deadly Sin

> *You don't have to be great to get started,*
> *but you have to get started to be great.*
>
> *- Les Brown*

Time management is another essential skill for nursing school success. We've already covered the first step towards effective time management - maintaining a daily planner. If you keep the planner updated and refer to it each night, half the battle is won. But now that you have all your projects, tests and assignments lined up, how to you prioritize them? Which items should you tackle first?

Prioritizing means putting things in order of importance. The most time-sensitive projects generally need more of your attention than less critical items. However, putting everything off until they *become* critical is not productive. Here's how to get a handle on things when you find yourself juggling multiple priorities and deadlines:

+ **Make a List**

    Make a quick list of everything on your plate - projects, exams, reading assignments, etc. Be sure to also include items of a personal nature you need to get done (i.e. renew car tags, file taxes, etc.).

+ **Rank 'em**

    Rank your to-do list items in order of importance. You can star the critical items, number them, or use a color-code system: red for critical, orange for items due in the near future, yellow for items not due for several weeks.

+ **Divide to conquer**

    Large projects need to be broken down into smaller chunks, to keep them from being overwhelming. Break things down into more manageable parts.

+ **Set mini-goals and deadlines**

    After breaking things into smaller chunks, set mini-goals (ex: rough draft done in two weeks). A little bit here, a little bit there - before you know it, you've got everything done.

+ **Stick to your plan**

    Keep up with your mini-goals and many a crisis will be averted. It's much easier to *choose* to work on something, than to *have* to work on something because it is due tomorrow.

Sometimes, no matter how hard you try, you just can't seem to get motivated. In fact, getting started is 90% of the battle. Personal trainers often advise clients who have trouble getting started to simply put on workout clothes. They know if clients can just get dressed for a workout, they are 10 times more likely to exercise that day, even if they don't feel like it.

The same principle applies here. If you can't seem to get started, make a deal with yourself. Agree to sit down with your materials for just 5 minutes. After that, you are free to get up, leave the work and do something else. Promise yourself that 5 minutes. 90% of the time, you'll go ahead and stick it out for a full study/homework session.

Procrastination is a chronic version of the "I-just-can't-seem-to-get-going- on-this" problem. There are deeper issues at work in procrastination than a momentary lack of commitment. Common reasons for procrastination include:

+ **I don't know how.**

    If you don't have all the tools or knowledge to complete an assignment, you may not even attempt it. If this pops up, don't let it be a stumbling block. Seek out the answers you need.

✦ **I have so much to do, I don't know where to begin!**
It's natural to feel overwhelmed sometimes, but if you feel this way most of the time, you may have a problem prioritizing and setting clear goals. Make a list and start with one thing at a time. Check off things you have completed so you can visually see the progress you are making.

✦ **What if I fail? What if I succeed?**
This kind of pressure can drive a person crazy. Some are afraid to try and fail, while others are afraid of doing too good a job, creating higher expectations for the next assignment. Try not to let negative self-talk get in the way of your goals. Take satisfaction in knowing you did your best - regardless of the grade.

> ### Giving Up Quality Time
> For me, the hardest part about nursing school was giving up quality time with family and friends in order to study for exams and master clinical skills.
> - Emily B. Horne, 2001 graduate
> Sampson Community College

The most important thing to remember when you face the procrastination monster is to take things one step at a time. Keep moving forward, even in tiny increments. The psychological lift you get from progress, no matter how small, will keep propelling you further.

Don't Forget

Keep your eye on the end result - don't get so overwhelmed with the details that you forget about the bigger picture. Every step, no matter how small, puts you that much closer to your goal.

Chicken Scratch

Taking good notes is not just a skill...it's an art form. There you sit, trying to listen to the instructor, process information and write it down, all at the same time. This makes patting your head while rubbing your tummy in a circular motion look easy.

First, let's look at the importance of notes. Why bother with them? In truth, there are a good number of students who don't take notes at all, preferring to actively listen and absorb the lecture content. But note taking, done correctly, can provide you with a highly targeted study and review guide. Putting things into your own words assists with comprehension and memory. For many people, taking notes also serves to help them stay focused in class (and who among us here has not drifted off during a particularly lengthy lecture?).

If you've ever borrowed notes from someone in your class, you know there are *good* note takers, and there are *not-so-good* note takers. The good note takers aren't just gifted at birth - they apply technique. There are ways you can make sure your notes are relevant, useful and legible (after all, if you can't read them later on - what good are they?).

The first thing good note takers learn is how to pick out the important stuff. Even if you are proficient at shorthand, you can't possibly write down every single word your teacher says. An astute student recognizes that instructors almost always give clues about what is important. Watch for the following during your lectures, which precede or indicate important information:

◆ Introductory phrases and summary statements.
◆ A big pause or added vocal emphasis.
◆ Anything written on the chalk board or overhead.
◆ Information that has been repeated several times.
◆ Questions to the class.
◆ Listing (i.e., "The top three reasons antibiotics are becoming resistant are...").

Tip

Once you have gotten the hang of "hearing" what's important, you can add some finesse to your notes. Here are some ways to make note taking easier and more efficient:

◆ **DO use consistent abbreviations**
Develop your own shorthand method for common words and phrases (i.e., treatment = Tx). Drop vowels or word endings (i.e., communication = commun; people = ppl).
◆ **DO make things stand out**
Use a star or exclamation point next to really important information. Circle things or highlight them.
◆ **DO divide the page**
Draw an off-center line down each page, just to the right of the margin. Write lecture notes on the right side of the line. Use the left side to add in details you missed later on.
◆ **DO streamline your notes**
Write your notes in outline form (main topic, principal ideas, sub-topics), or use flowcharts/idea maps. Draw pictures and make lists.
◆ **DON'T write in complete sentences.**
◆ **DON'T get hung up on grammar and spelling.**
◆ **DON'T try to write down every word.**

Watch Out

Try to capture all the main points, then the subpoints. If it's allowed, use a tape recorder to record your lectures. Play back the tape as you go over your notes and fill in anything you missed.

Tip

If at all possible, tape record the very first lecture -you will be thrown a lot of information in the first class meeting, and being human, you will miss some of it. Play the tape back later that evening to catch important information you missed the first time around.

A few final thoughts on note taking - be sure to review your notes as soon as possible after class. This helps reinforce the material in your mind. And if you miss a lecture, borrow two sets of notes to copy from. This will increase your chances of getting a complete overview of what was covered in class.

Study Groups

Study groups are the backbone of nursing school. With study groups, you can cover more material faster by evenly distributing a heavy workload. A good study group offers you the chance to develop and improve teamwork, leadership, teaching and problem-solving skills. Additionally, it provides you with a support system. *Nursing school is a cooperative experience - not a competitive one -* and students are called upon to share and teach what they are learning.

For a study group to be effective, it needs to follow a couple of guidelines:
+ Limit the size of the group to 4 or 5 people maximum.
+ Meet at the same time and place on a regular basis.
+ Work together to develop a mission statement for the group, expressing common goals and intentions.
+ Agree on work time - socializing and fun occurs at the *end* of the meeting.
+ Divide the work evenly - everyone needs to pull an equal amount of weight.

Using the course syllabus is a good way to develop common goals for the group - what are the expected outcomes of the course? What can the group do together to meet those objectives?

What exactly do study groups do? They outline reading assignments, research medical information, study for exams and quiz each other. They compare notes, work on projects, give feedback, divide work and share experiences. They tutor, mentor, support and motivate each other. Your study group will do all these things and more, adapting to the ever-changing needs and focus of the group.

A Guided Tour of Your Classes

You've made the big time...real nursing classes. Exhilarating isn't it? You're probably just a teensy bit curious about the classes you will be taking and what to expect.

In this section, we'll take a peek at the most common nursing courses to give you an idea of what you will be learning. I've also included a short list of the basic prerequisite courses. But first, let's dispel (or confirm, as the case may be) some of the more prevalent nursing school myths...

Nursing School Horror Stories

You've all heard the rumors - whispered in the halls by nervous new students, or proclaimed with undeniable certainty by upper classmen:

A friend of a friend whose sister's brother-in-law was in nursing school 2 years ago said they each had to manage 15 patients all by themselves in clinicals.

A former student at the college, who was kicked out for having a sloppy uniform, read in the paper that a patient in Arizona died when students practicing IV therapy hung the wrong meds.

A student's neighbor's best friend's uncle said he saw a student get sucked into the MRI machine by her eyebrow piercing.

Urban legends - you've got to love 'em.

Don't Panic

Most of the stories you hear are only *partially* true, if that. And by the way, none of the above scenarios has one bit of truth to them (whew!). Take everything you hear with a grain of salt. The bottom line is, you will never be required to do anything you haven't been trained for yet, and until you have proven yourself, you will never be left to fly solo.

To be fair, some things are true, if only partially so:

MYTH?
Nursing school instructors are merciless drill sergeants intent on making you drop out.

This all depends on your frame of reference. Nursing school instructors are hardly heartless - remember, they went into the field for the same reasons you did - and they have dedicated themselves to teaching and mentoring the next generation of nurses. They do not want you to drop out - to the contrary, they want you to *succeed.*

Nursing school is hard and a lot will be expected of you. You will be pushed to learn and do more than you ever imagined possible. When your instructors are hard on you, it is for your own benefit (Really! You'll be glad for it later). They have been charged with helping you develop all the skills necessary to become a nurse. Mistakes by nurses *and* nursing students can cost patients their lives. Nursing instructors HAVE to be hard on you - to do otherwise would be a grave disservice to you, and dangerous for the public.

MYTH?

If you don't score 100% on your drug dosage test, you will be dropped from the program.

In many schools, yes - this is true. This also applies to a few other tests, such as your physical assessment skills test. Some programs require a score of 90%, others require only that you pass, and still others require a perfect score. Either way, if you do not meet the required grade, you certainly can be dropped from the program. That's a reality.

The good news is this will not come as a surprise. You will be told ahead of time if the test is an all-or-nothing, win-or-lose exam. If you know ahead of time, you can prepare. You can study. You can practice. You can do it! If it was impossible, we wouldn't have any nurses, right? Right!

MYTH?

You have to practice giving injections on each other.

Also true, depending on your particular program. But you will not be handed a needle on the first day and be expected to start poking people. You will practice on lab dummies first, and sometimes even oranges. Only when you have a good amount of practice and confidence will you be moved on to live subjects. For those of you who are needle-phobic, take heart - your instructors will work with you.

Core Classes

Every nursing program has its own unique curriculum designed to provide you with the knowledge base and skills-set necessary to become a good nurse. You will find, however, that there are some courses common to all nursing programs. The names may vary, but you can expect to take the following core classes in nursing school. *Note that this represents a typical BSN curriculum; ADN programs will be similar, but with less prerequisites, and LPN programs follow a condensed curriculum that will be significantly different.*

The Prerequisites

The complete list applies to BSN programs. Typical ADN prerequisites have are designated with an asterisk (*):

College Algebra*

Statistics

Biology*

Anatomy*

Chemistry*

Physiology*

Microbiology

Nutrition

English Composition I & II*

Public Speaking

Psychology*

Developmental Psychology

Sociology

History

Humanities Electives (i.e., Philosophy, Art, etc.)

Watch Out

Notice that the prerequisites are heavy on the science and math courses - while you should not let this intimidate you, you should be prepared to devote extra time to your studies for these classes. The science courses, in particular, require more time, but they are also worth more credit hours, so it's a fair trade. To keep your sanity, it's wise to take no more than 2 science courses per semester.

NURSING CLASSES

Foundations in Nursing

This will be one of the very first nursing courses you take. *Foundations in Nursing* introduces the basic concepts and principles around which nursing practice is built. The class will give you an overview of nursing care, theory, primary patient needs, standards and the healthcare system. You will also learn how economic, historical, technological and legal issues influence nursing practice.

Health Promotion/Assessment Skills

Physical exam, patient assessment, vital signs and documentation of historical data are covered in this class through hands-on lab work. Additionally, you will learn to design developmentally appropriate methods of promoting and maintaining health, and will be taught basic care skills (such as bathing, transferring, assisting with personal hygiene, etc.).

Pathophysiology

Pathophysiology focuses on the biological processes that can be altered by human disease (basically, what happens when we get sick). Here you will learn to distinguish the various clinical manifestations of the disease process.

Pharmacology

Remember how difficult anatomy was, memorizing 2400 different body parts? *Pharmacology* is the same way - not impossible obviously, but it will be intense. You will learn about basic concepts and theories in pharmacology, major drug classifications, nutritional supplements and the role pharmacology plays in nursing.

Therapeutic Interventions

This course will help you develop the skills and techniques necessary to apply therapeutic interventions. Included will be time management techniques, effective delegation, prioritization skills, team building, drug calculations and cost control concepts.

Community Health Nursing

The role of the nurse in the community and issues affecting the health of society are covered in this course. Emphasis is placed on the promotion of public health.

Intercultural Nursing

This course introduces methods for effective delivery of care to patients of various cultures, backgrounds and belief systems.

Nursing Ethics

Nursing Ethics is designed to facilitate the clarification of personal values, while fostering ethical decision-making in the nursing profession. Critical thinking and effective analysis of ethical issues will be stressed.

Nursing Research

This is an introductory course to the basic elements of research. You will be familiarized with statistical methods, critical analysis of data and standard terminology.

Leadership/Management in Nursing

As the title implies, this course develops leadership and management skills for use in nursing practice. Individual, group and organizational dynamics, conflict resolution, legal issues and work-related stress are covered.

And that's not all! You will have other courses not mentioned here, including advanced levels of the nursing foundations and assessment classes. Don't forget there will also be clinicals, which run concurrently with your lecture courses and labs.

Don't Panic

It sounds like a lot, but it will never be more than you can handle. The curriculum is designed so that coursework and clinicals complement each other. Each new skill will be built on previously learned skills, the end result being a well-rounded, thorough education in nursing practice.

Front and Center: In the Classroom

A child comes home from his first day of school. His mother asks, "Well, what did you learn today?" The kid replies, "Not enough. They want me to come back again tomorrow."

By now you are very familiar with the college lecture course. The teacher stands up in front of the class and lectures while you take notes. Everything is outlined for you ahead of time, so you know what will be covered when. Classes are typically good-sized, and if you are absent, you might not even be missed.

Nursing lecture courses, however, are a little different. For one thing, your lecture course may not involve any lectures at all. You may be given reading assignments to study on your own time, while during class, you are instructed in skills. Or, alternatively, you might find yourself in a lecture class with only 5 to 7 people. You will be expected to *participate*. You will also be called on to think critically and draw conclusions without your teaching spelling it out for you. These are upper-level courses - you will not be spoon-fed.

As a nursing student, you will be treated as a mature adult. You will be solely responsible for your own choices and actions. No one will tell you that you need to do your homework or you need to be in class. It is expected that you will do so, because you *chose* to be in the program. It is also expected that you will participate, ask questions if you need clarification on something and seek help when you need it. The burden is on you to be proactive in advocating for your needs.

The following sections offer tips to help you flourish in the rich nursing school lecture environment. Advice for getting the most out of your classes includes information on collegial sharing, public speaking, term papers and managing the enormous volume of information you will be expected to learn. Oh yes...and how to figure out your professor's modus operandi...

Identify Your Instructor's Style

I am always ready to learn, but I do not always like being taught.
- Sir Winston Churchill

Identifying your instructor's personal teaching style goes a long way towards succeeding in class. If you understand how they work, you will be better prepared for the types of exams they will give and what they expect from you in class.

Listen very carefully during the first class meeting, paying close attention to body language. Are they approachable? Authoritarian? Dramatic? Closed-Off? How do they interact with students?

If your teacher is very well-organized, you had better be, too! If they love to cite facts and figures, study the details in your notes and text. If they wax poetic about theories, expect to write some essays in the near future. The more you know about your instructors' personal preferences, the better insight you have into their expectations of you.

Tip

A good tip here is to talk to upper classmen - ask for feedback on your instructors. Your fellow nursing students will be a font of valuable information. Of course, you still have to do your work to pass any class - knowing your teacher's style doesn't mean you know your material - but it sure is helpful to have words of advice from students who have been there!

You will have all kinds of professors in nursing school, each sharing with you their own personal strengths and unique teaching abilities. Love 'em or hate 'em, you will most certainly *learn* from them, and that's what you are there for.

While every instructor is unique, sometimes you can't help but to draw generalized conclusions about certain "types" of teachers. In keeping with this time-honored tradition, here is a humorous, tongue-in-cheek look at some of the teachers you may encounter...see if you recognize any!

THE 4ᵀᴴ HORSEMAN OF THE APOCALYPSE (AKA MR. ARMAGEDDON)

You know you have Mr. Armageddon in the first 5 minutes of class - he is the one who starts his introduction with, *"50% of the people enrolled in my course will drop. Of the remaining 50%, half will fail. I have only given out one A in the last 10 years."* How's that for a hello? Don't let him psych you out. His bark is worse than his doom-and-gloom bite. To get through this course, you will need to keep on top of things. No waiting until the last minute to cram for an exam - it won't be possible. Exams are most likely multiple choice and matching - the matching questions will be the worst. You'll have to keep yourself motivated...he's not a pat-you-on-the-back kind of guy, so a study group is ideal for this class. One final note: As he beginneth, so will he endeth. You can bet your last $5 that sometime before finals, he will pronounce, *"The final is comprehensive and worth 35% of your grade. It is not uncommon for students to drop one to two letter grades because of the final..."*

THE MARTHA STEWART PROTEGÉ

The Martha Stewart Protegé is one very thorough lady. She has learning objectives and a comprehensive course outline neatly spiral-bound for you. She has a web site with lecture notes, practice exams and supplementary links at your disposal. She has handouts, practice exercises and study guides to give you, and if need be, a tutor waiting in the wings. Our gal Martha is very efficient and organized.

She put a lot of time into developing these resource materials, and she expects you to use them. There will be no excuses in this class for failing, after all the help she has made available to you. Expect the exams to have concrete true/false, multiple choice and equation-solving questions. Know your facts - the tests inevitably end up being harder than you expect.

THE STORYTELLER

The Storyteller *loves* to pepper her lectures with personal stories and anecdotes. Always entertaining, and often fascinating to listen to, the Storyteller adds depth and dimension to lecture materials through the use of real-life examples. Storytellers tend to pack a lot of information into their courses and keep up a fast, lively pace. If you have a Storyteller, the key thing to remember is *application*. Just as the Storytellers have applied the material to first-hand case scenarios for illustration purposes, so will you be expected to apply what you have learned during exams. Expect multiple choice questions that pull information together from many different areas, requiring applied knowledge and critical thinking. Storytellers also heavily favor essay questions and pop quizzes.

BUELLER...? BUELLER...? BUELLER...?

"The role of the teacher is - anyone? Anyone? To provide inforMAtion... information so you can - anyone? Anyone? Learn. So you can learn. The purpose of which is to - anyone? Anyone? Give you an edu-CA-tion..."

OK, this teacher is not going to win any personality contests, or the Most Innovative Teacher of the Year Award, but he's a good guy, just trying to do his job. We all have a Bueller professor at one time or another - it's inevitable. The Bueller's lectures are monotone and devoid of any life...paying attention may be the biggest challenge in his class. But let's have a little reality check here. *You* are paying to get an education. *You* are the one who chose to become a nurse. It is *your* job to take the information you are given and learn it. Sure, it's fun when we have a lively or humorous teacher, but it is *not* the teacher's job to entertain us. It is *not* the teacher's job to motivate us or hold our interest. The teacher is in charge of giving us the information we need, while we are in charge of motivating ourselves and learning it. So...suck it up, go to class and learn, even if it IS boring. Oh yes, and his testing style - anyone? Anyone? Fill-in-the-blank, of course!

Learning Objectives

Learning objectives - what are they anyway? Included in the course syllabus for each of your classes will be a list of learning objectives. These are the things you will be expected to know by the end of the term. Follow the line of logic here...if you are expected to know these things by the end of the semester, it stands to reason that you will be tested on them *during* the semester. If objectives 1 through 5 are covered in the first unit, it stands to reason that you will be tested on them in the first unit exam. Right? Right! So...the learning objectives can easily be used as a handy study guide for each of your tests. Nifty, huh?

To turn your objectives into a study guide, flip them around into questions. For example:

<u>Learning Objective #1:</u>
Students will be able to perform metric conversions and will be able recognize standard units of measure.

Becomes…

<u>Study Guide Questions for Objective #1:</u>
- ◆ How do you convert pounds to grams? Milligrams to kilograms?
- ◆ What is the abbreviation for milliliters? Cubic centimeters?
- ◆ What are conversion factors? How do they work?

Make up as many questions as you can for each objective. Use these questions to quiz yourself and study for exams. The learning objectives will give you the big picture - the framework from within which you can develop a plan of attack to learn the *right* things.

Taking it All in

> *Your grade point average is not important,*
> *It's the amount of your learning.*
>
> *- Ravindra Bansal*

As noted earlier, showing up for class consistently is certainly a great first step to doing well in school. *Absorbing* all the information in lectures, however, does tend to require more effort.

To truly benefit from your lectures, you need to employ *active listening*. Hearing is passive - the spoken word floats into your ear without effort or direction from you. Active listening on the other hand is, well…active. It is the self-initiated process of trying to understand what is being said. Active listening means getting to the heart of the message being sent and identifying its applicability within the framework of the bigger picture.

There are several things you can do to help create the right mental atmosphere for active listening:

Tip

- ✦ Read up ahead of time on the material to be covered, so you will be familiar with the information.
- ✦ Come to class well-rested, wearing comfortable clothing.
- ✦ Arrive on time.
- ✦ Sit as close to the front as possible - you'll pay more attention.

During the lecture, stay on target. The following tips will help you further develop your active listening skills:

- ✦ Always keep the main idea of the lecture in the forefront of your mind.
- ✦ Rephrase things in your own words while taking notes.
- ✦ Keep your focus - if you find your mind wandering, rein it back in.
- ✦ Ask questions.
- ✦ Participate in class discussions.

Following these tips will help you pay attention to and absorb the material being presented.

When you are learning something new, the information is automatically stored in your short-term memory. Your goal is to get it moved to your long term memory, so it will set up permanent residence. The problem is, as a general rule, the new stuff isn't allowed into the long term memory without an escort.

If you can connect the new information to something you already know, two things happen: First, the thing-you-already-know pops out of your long term memory and goes to see what all the ruckus is in your short term memory. This is known as *recalling* information - you are calling it out of storage.

Once in your short term memory again, the thing-you-already-know meets up with the new information. They hang out together and become instant friends - they "click." When the party's over and it's time to go home, the thing-you-already-know takes the new information with it. And THAT is how you learn something so it sticks.

When in class, try to link the information you are currently learning to a concept or piece of information you already know. That will give the new information a free one-way ticket to your long term memory.

Reading with a Purpose

I know God will not give me anything I can't handle.
I just wish He didn't trust me so much.

- Mother Teresa

Okay, you have 40 different text and reference books, three binders full of handouts and five steno pads' worth of notes - front *and* back. The little guys in your long term memory are threatening to unionize and go on strike, while your short term memory admissions clerk has hung a "No Vacancy" sign.

What do you do when you face overwhelming amounts of information? How do you sort through it all? And more importantly, how are you going to remember it all?

We've already discussed ways to prioritize the work and break it down so it is more manageable. Even so, it may still feel like the odds are stacked against you - after all, there are only 24 hours in a day, most of which are already consumed by school, outside responsibilities and the occasional full night of sleep.

One solution could be to take up speed reading - you would certainly be able to cover more material! But would your remember any of it? Hard to say. A more effective technique would be *active reading*.

Just as there is a distinction between hearing and active listening, there is also a difference between leisurely reading and *active reading*. Leisurely reading is done purely for enjoyment. This is what we are used to. Leisurely reading is great, but when you have 400 pages of heavy medical text to get through, enjoyment is the farthest thing from your mind. What happens here is that our minds balk. "Hey...this is not *fun* - we're outta here!"

Active reading, on the other hand, is *reading with a mission*. Instead of sitting down to read, we sit down to find out something in particular. Our mind no longer balks, because our focus has shifted from reading to hunting. It's semantics, obviously...but the distinction trick works.

Try this the next time you have to wade through a technical chapter. Skim the headings, like we discussed earlier, and ask yourself, "What do I want to know after having read this chapter?" Your mind will pop to attention and immediately start seeking the answers as you read. You will read faster as your mind hunts for the target information, skimming the fluff and diving straight for the meat.

Ask and Ye Shall Be Answered

Imagine you are the instructor. You are giving a two-hour lecture on some pretty complex material that is vital for your students to understand. While you speak, everyone sits in silence, smiling and nodding politely. The only sound other than your voice is that of pens furiously scribbling away.

As you move deeper into the subject material, your students' eyes begin to glaze over. From the sea of blank stares, you realize you might as well be talking about lawn maintenance. Is anyone getting the information? Are you going too fast? Is anyone even listening or did you mistakenly walk into the Stepford Wives convention?

Teachers rely on student feedback to gauge classroom progress towards learning goals. They need you to let them know what more you need, so they can facilitate your learning. Asking questions is vital.

People tend to get shy when it comes to the question-asking thing. Some feel they are wasting class time, or worry about what others will think. Nonsense! Your questions are valid and worthy of being asked - period. You absolutely have a right to ask questions. It is *your* education, after all, so if you don't understand something, ask! The smart student is not the one who has no questions - he is the one who has the initiative to ask for answers.

If you need more convincing, think on this: 99% of the time that you don't quite get something, or are confused about a concept, there will be at least two other people (often more) who are wondering exactly the same thing. They will be glad you asked, your teacher will be glad you asked, and in the end, *you* will be glad you asked, because you will have your answers.

Ask

A final thought: before you can learn to advocate for patients, you have to learn to advocate for yourself. When in doubt, ask, ask, ask!

Your Two Cents - It Counts!

True classroom participation goes beyond just asking questions - participation means getting *involved* in the discussions, sharing thoughts and ideas. Participation gives you ownership of what you are learning.

This is an important concept to understand because taking ownership of your learning represents a shift in thinking. You go from passive learner presented with things to do (I *have* to do this), to active learner and seeker of knowledge (I *choose* to do this, because it is the most efficient way to reach my goals). You become a co-creator of the educational process and are empowered to learn.

It always comes as a surprise to hear students complaining about assignments or how demanding their teachers are, or worse, that they are expected to learn too much. These students have not taken ownership of their education - they are still stuck in the mindset that lets them believe someone is making them do things they don't want to do.

Are we not all adults by the time we are in college? Are we not there for a specific purpose? No one is forcing this education on you. Understanding this will help you get away from a dependent parent-child mentality to a more independent view of the educator-student relationship.

When you take ownership of your education, you will find you are free to contribute to discussions and participate in class. The more you contribute, the more you will get out of each lecture.

Don't Forget

Remember this, to start you on the right path, you have permission to:
   ✦ Think for yourself.
   ✦ Develop your own opinions.
   ✦ Investigate, question and learn to your heart's content.
Participate in class; open yourself up to personal growth. A true education goes beyond the books, and through classroom participation, you guarantee yourself the most enriching educational experience possible.

The Art of Public Speaking

> *It's alright to have butterflies in your stomach.*
> *Just get them to fly in formation.*
>
> *- Dr. Rob Gilbert*

What is the number-one phobia in America? Fear of heights? Fear of snakes? Fear of flying? No, the most common phobia we have is the fear of giving a speech. Something about standing up in front of a group of people makes our blood run cold and fills us with dread. Just the thought of giving a speech is enough to cause our hearts to pound and our breathing rates to skyrocket.

Good public speaking skills are essential for nurses - think patient/family education, communication with peers and clients, and health presentations in the community. As daunting as it seems now, you will be glad for the training later.

Short of hypnotherapy or faking an illness, is there help to be had? Of course there is. The answer lies in thorough preparation and practice. The better you prepare, the more confident you will be. The more you practice, the less frightening it will seem.

When you are developing a presentation, you want to make sure you know your topic inside and out. Read as much as you can and do your research. When you have developed the right knowledge-base, you can go on to create a fantastic presentation.

There are certain things you will want to keep in mind as you prepare your presentation:

- ✦ Follow instructions - make sure you meet the guidelines set by your instructor (i.e., only two points, 10 minutes maximum, etc.).
- ✦ Limit yourself to three main points unless otherwise directed.
- ✦ Use supporting details, but don't get lost in them - keep the focus on the main points.
- ✦ Give an overview of what your speech will be about at the beginning, and summarize at the end.
- ✦ Don't get too technical - use common language.
- ✦ Keep sentences short and concise.
- ✦ Write with your time limit in mind.

You know from experience that sitting through a speech or lecture can be tedious. As a speaker, you need to think of ways to keep your audience's attention. Common techniques for spicing up a speech include:

- ✦ Visual aids (charts, graphs, pictures).
- ✦ Humor.
- ✦ Personal anecdotes.
- ✦ Interesting or thought-provoking facts and trivia.

Tip

The key here is not to overdo it. As with fashion, less is more. Using a few of these items at appropriate intervals will help keep your audience alert, without over-stimulating them.

Once you have written your speech, practice it. Then, practice it some more. Pay special attention to transitions from one part of the speech to the next. Memorizing these so you can recite them on a moment's notice will help you move on if you get lost while giving the speech.

When you are given an oral presentation assignment, you are often not given any guidelines or advice on *how* to give your speech. Researching and writing a speech is one thing - actually presenting it is another. While there are countless schools of thought on what makes a good speaker, there are some basic techniques you can adopt fairly easily to polish your presentation skills.

The first thing to remember is that your image is almost as important as the speech itself. Dress appropriately for the audience and pay attention to personal grooming. It will enhance your credibility and effectiveness as a speaker.

Pay attention to your non-verbal communication. Stand tall, feet slightly apart, head up. Keep your hands open, so the palms show. Make eye-contact with audience members and smile from time to time. Use gestures that feel comfortable to you and avoid pointing at the audience. Above all, be confident, or at the very least, pretend you are (sometimes this works just as well).

More techniques you can use to polish your presentation:
- Lower the tone of your voice.
- Slow down your speed - breathe slower, speak slower, use pauses.
- Project your voice to the back of the room and speak clearly.
- If you are using visual aids, point to them when you are speaking about them.
- Take three steps toward the audience when making an important point.
- For large crowds, use larger, slower gestures.
- For more intimate crowds, use smaller, quicker gestures.

And what of speech no-no's? There are some things you should avoid at all costs, primarily because they detract from your credibility.

Tip

The Seven Deadly Sins of Oral Presentation
1. Keeping your hands in your pockets.
2. Clenching your fists.
3. Putting your hands on your hips or in front of you in the "fig leaf" position.
4. Fidgeting.
5. Mistaking shouting for projecting.
6. Statue Syndrome - being afraid to move at all.
7. Running way over or under your time limit.

Work on your presentation until it feels like second nature. The more comfortable you are with it ahead of time, the better you will feel during the actual presentation.

Additionally, some people like to use cue cards in case they forget something, but take care if you choose to go this route. Sometimes, using cue cards as back-up only serves to fluster you more when you lose your place and have to search for the right spot on the right card. In my experience, it's better to memorize your speech solidly and get in enough rehearsal ahead of time so you can proceed with confidence.

Don't Forget

Finally, the public speaking skills that you are acquiring and practicing will be quite useful in your career. Remember the "big picture."

The Written Word

Don't use a big word where a diminutive word will suffice.

- Anonymous

Writing plays a large role in nursing. The ability to effectively communicate your patient's condition and needs on paper is critical to ensuring the continuity of care. Documentation is an ongoing requirement of the job, and as a member of a professional team, you will often be called on to communicate with administration and peers via the written medium.

As a student, you will write term papers, essays, care plans and more. Paying attention to your writing now will serve you well in the future (and help your grades, to boot!). Just as public speaking is an acquired skill, so is effective writing. The goal is to communicate your point in the most concise, clear manner possible, without glaring errors that detract from the message.

Some basic rules apply to all written assignments:

- ✦ Clarity is essential - your readers must be able to understand what you are saying.
- ✦ Spelling and grammar counts - always.
- ✦ Neatness is a must - unless it's on an exam, type everything.

That said, there are some guidelines you can follow to increase the effectiveness of your writing:

Tip

Ten Tips for Better Writing

1. Narrow your focus

Whether you are writing an essay or a research paper, make sure your topic is as narrow as possible (i.e., instead of "The History of Nursing," write about "Civil War Nursing.").

2. Define your audience

Who are you writing for? Your instructor? Your classmates? A scholarship committee? Keep your audience in mind as you structure your paper.

3. Organize your work

Outline your essay or paper first and build a coherent, logical progression from beginning to end.

4. Introduce and summarize

Always give an overview of the contents of your paper at the beginning and a summary paragraph at the end.

5. Use transitions

Don't jump from one idea to the next without a transition. Connect the two so the information flows logically.

6. Be concise
Say what you mean to say. Don't worry about flowery fluff, just state things as directly as possible.

7. Use an active voice
The active voice has more power than the passive voice:
Passive: The patient was given meds by the nurse on duty.
Active: The nurse on duty gave the patient meds.

8. Add variety
Vary the length of your sentences and their structure. Use synonyms to avoid repetition.

9. Avoid getting too familiar
The words "you" and "I" should be avoided unless specifically appropriate for your audience and message.

10. Write to express, not to impress
Filling your paper with big, impressive words adds nothing to your credibility. Keep it simple.

Tip

Another thing I would recommend is investing in the *American Psychological Association (APA) Publication Manual.* More than likely, all of your nursing papers will have to follow the specific format outlined in this style guide

As you are writing, you may get stuck. It may be that you can't quite get a transition to work the way you'd like, or you may just have plain old Writer's Block, with no idea where to go next. In either case, the best thing to do is to take a quick break and revisit your writing in 10 minutes. If you still find you are stuck, free form. Just start writing. Ideas will come to you as you initiate movement.

When you have finished your paper, proof it for errors. Don't rely solely on your spell checker. A trick secretaries use to catch mistakes is to proofread backwards, starting with the last word first. It is also very helpful to have others proof your paper. They will catch errors you have missed.

Watch Out

It should go without saying, but plagiarism is a big no-no -nursing schools don't treat this issue lightly. All your work needs to be your own, and your sources must be cited and credited appropriately.

Don't Panic

A special note on charting - there is a special lingo used in charting, a nursing language, which will be unfamiliar at first. Don't worry if everything looks Greek - you will master it in no time. The key to "getting" it is simply repetition and consistent use (and believe me, you'll get all the practice you need!).

Effective writing is a skill that does take time to learn, but as with any craft, the more practice you get, the better you will be. Remember, top-notch communication skills (*including* the written kind) are essential to your nursing career - which is why it plays such a big part in your education.

Anxiety-Free Exams

Once upon a time, there was an ant and a grasshopper...

"Wait a minute!" you say, "We've heard this story already. The little ant works all summer long finding and storing food for the winter while the grasshopper plays. Yadda, yadda, yadda, winter comes, the ant is toasty warm and well-fed, while the grasshopper dies of starvation and frostbite. Moral of the story, don't put things off until it's too late, right?"

Well...sort of. You're not far off. But this ant and grasshopper story is a little different. To continue...

Once upon a time there was an ant and a grasshopper... and a duck-billed platypus.

Caught you off-guard there with the platypus, didn't I?

The ant and the platypus were both in nursing school together. The grasshopper, in case you were wondering, had too much fun partying his freshman year and dropped out of college before even applying to the nursing program.

Moving on...

The ant was a very diligent student - borderline obsessive-compulsive, if you ask me. He worked tirelessly night and day, faithfully completing every reading assignment, practice exercise and "Test Your Knowledge" question at chapter's end. He could recite the medical dictionary verbatim. In fact, he was a walking encyclopedia of nursing knowledge and people were awed by his presence.

The duck-billed platypus, on the other hand, was an average student with an above-average desire to be a good nurse. She budgeted her time so she could study and keep up with the material, but she also included time for herself. She developed relationships with her classmates and instructors. She participated in lively class discussions about ethics and patient-centered care. She observed nurses in action during clinicals, and spent time just talking with her patients. She never was too busy to lend an ear to a distraught classmate, nor was she so focused on grades that she ever forgot her <u>real</u> purpose in school - to understand what she was being taught and how it applied to real-life situations.

"Hmmm, okay...great for the platypus - she's a team player. But the ant is obviously going to do better on his exams, right?"

Not so, young grasshopper (I've been dying to work that line into this book somehow...).

The day of the first major exam finally came. The ant, extremely cranky from lack of sleep, arrogantly strolled into class and announced he would be the first person to ever get an "A" from Mr. Armageddon. Everyone ignored him.

The platypus came in smiling (she had gotten a full night's sleep and was feeling downright perky). She wished everyone good luck and mentally prepared to begin the exam.

The test was handed out and everyone in class began silently working on it. The ant caught his breath and muttered, stunned, "WHAT? What IS this?" You see, this test did not ask for facts and figures. It presented case scenarios and asked students to think critically. It required them to apply the facts they had learned to case situations, taking into consideration the needs of the patients and their families. The ant turned red, started to shake violently, and finally, exploded. All that remained was a pile of dust.

"Wow, that was pretty graphic."

The platypus, on the other hand, used what she had learned from her text and lectures, as well as what she had learned from interacting with her instructors, other students, nurses and patients. She was a student of humanity, as well as a student of nursing. She did not get an "A" from Mr. Armageddon, but she did get a well-deserved "B." And after the exam, she was invited to go out and celebrate with her classmates.

"Cute...and the moral of the story is...?"

We were hoping you would ask. The moral of the story is:

Don't Forget

> *Don't be so focused on grades that you forget the big picture.*
> *If you cannot apply the information you have learned, you will be lost.*

You see, test-taking is not about getting an "A"; rather, exams are a tool to assess your progress. Use them to help you define your weak areas. Learn from them. Remember, he who graduates last in his class gets the same diploma as he who graduates first.

The main idea is that you want to leave nursing school with a thorough enough knowledge base and skills-set to do your job well. Focus on this, not the letter grade - and you will succeed. As a bonus, good grades will naturally follow -which by the way are important for some scholarships and for graduate school.

Now, if we have your promise to not obsess about grades, we'll share strategies to help you prepare for exams and a few techniques you can use to improve your scores. But you're not going to obsess, you promised - right? Right! Okay then...

Strategies for Test Prep

You know you need to show up for class and study as you go - that's the only *real* way to do it if you want guaranteed peace of mind the night before an exam. But in the real world, things happen. Sometimes, we are not able to be as diligent as we would like. It's okay if this happens every now and again - don't beat yourself up about it. If, however, you find it happens constantly and you are feeling overwhelming the majority of the time, flip back to the sections on Organizational Skills and Procrastination for a quick review on prioritizing your life.

Also, another resource you have at your disposal is your school advisor or counselor. Seek them out for strategies and suggestions.

When you are studying for an exam, find a quiet place free of distractions. If this means leaving your house and setting up shop at the library or local bookstore, so be it. You need to be able to concentrate.

Things you can use to prepare for the test:
- ✦ Your notes from class - instructors test on what they teach.
- ✦ Your flashcards (you've been making them all along, right?).
- ✦ The learning objectives - make them into a study guide.
- ✦ Your text book and any supplementary handouts.
- ✦ One or two NCLEX prep books -they are broken down into subject areas you can use for class exams and will help with critical thinking, spotting weak areas and test taking. As an added bonus, you will be preparing for the big exam down the road.

Try to think of questions that will be on the exam, and make sure you know the answers. If you have already figured out your instructor's style, you are a step ahead of the game, as you can anticipate the kinds of questions he or she will most likely ask. If not, think back to the items stressed in class. What topics did the instructor spend the most time on?

A good strategy - if the information is not already obvious to you, is to go ahead and ask the instructor directly about the test format and level of difficulty. Hey, it can't hurt. Also, if possible, ask upperclassman about the kinds of tests your instructor gives.

Use your study group to prepare for the test. Five heads are better than one, right? With your group, go over as many different problems as you can. Quiz each other. If you don't know how to do something, ask a member to teach you. Likewise, if you notice another member struggling with a concept you understand, teach them. Try to keep the group on track for serious studying by planning breaks every 45 minutes. This will allow time for needed stress relief and help keep everyone focused on the task at hand.

Don't trick yourself into believing the old "I perform better under pressure" lie. Why make yourself crazy at the last minute? You'd be better off doing a little studying here and there ahead of time. If you find your back up against the wall and absolutely have to cram for an exam, make sure you learn the main points. Don't get lost in the details. You will do better overall knowing the big picture than knowing random, unconnected details.

Get plenty of rest the night before an exam. Staying up until 3 a.m. studying will actually have an adverse affect on your performance. You will most likely not retain the information you have crammed, and you will be less alert during the exam. In the same vein, take a few moments to eat breakfast - it will give you added energy to help you stay focused.

Pack your bag the night before with all the supplies you need - pencils, calculator, etc. To be on the safe side, set two alarms if you have them. Lay out your clothes to save time in the morning and make sure your car has gas so you will be ready to roll.

What's the Question?

There are several different kinds of exam questions - essay, multiple choice, fill-in-the-blank, etc. Usually, an exam will feature a combination of them. In every case, the most important thing you can do is to read the instructions and read the questions. It doesn't matter how much you know if you don't follow the rules. For example, you'll lose points on a "compare and contrast" short answer if you only note similarities and don't include differences. Make sure you know what the question is asking.

And now for some quick tips to get you through those exams!

Tip

General Advice

- ✦ Your first instinct is usually right. Avoid changing your answers unless you are certain you were wrong.
- ✦ If you can't remember something, circle it and come back. Many times, the information you need to jog your memory will appear in another question on the test.
- ✦ Scan the exam briefly at the outset - answer the easiest questions first.
- ✦ Review your test before turning it in. Check all your work for accuracy.

Multiple Choice

◆ **READ the question**

Underline qualifiers, such as "all," "none," and "most"

◆ **Narrow your choices**

There is usually at least one ridiculous answer you can throw out. Try to narrow your choices down to two answers, then make an educated guess.

◆ **When all else fails, the answer is "C"**

Oddly enough, this is true - C is the most often used letter for correct answers. If you are not penalized for guessing (i.e., if you don't earn negative points for answering incorrectly), and you have no idea what the answer is...go for C - it can't hurt.

Fill-In-The-Blank

◆ **Use the line length as your guide**

Oftentimes, the blank line will be longer when the correct answer is a long word. If there are two or three blanks, you know the correct answer has two or three terms, respectively.

◆ **Answer specifically what was asked**

Read the question carefully to determine what answer is expected.

◆ **Never leave it blank**

Write in something - it can't hurt, and sometimes you will surprise yourself.

True/False

◆ **Watch the qualifiers**

True/false questions with absolute qualifiers (such as "always," "never," "all" and "none") are most often false. Qualifiers such as "sometimes," "usually" and "most of the time" are typically true.

◆ **Stick to your guns**

So what if you have more "T's" than "F's" or vice versa? There is no rule saying there will be exactly the same number of true answers as false ones.

Essay

◆ **Answer the question first**

Make sure you put in the information directly asked for.

◆ **Add other details as time allows**

If time allows, fill out your essay with supporting details once the main objective has been met.

◆ **Pay attention to the specifics**

Make sure you include everything asked for, especially in multiple-part essay questions. Pay attention to instructions, such as "compare and contrast." Don't forget to answer the last part of a "describe how this works" question - it is almost always followed by "why?"

Budgeting Exam Time

An often overlooked ingredient to successful test-taking is budgeting your time wisely. Most tests have a time limit and if you don't keep tabs on the clock, you may run out of time.

Scan through the test when you receive it to give yourself an idea of the layout and difficulty-level of each section. Answer the easiest questions first, saving the hard ones for the end. This will assure you of more correct answers (and a higher score) if you run out of time.

In general, spend the first half of your allotted time working on the quick-answer questions (multiple choice, true/false, matching and fill-in-the-blank). The second half should be reserved for essay questions and math problems - there will be fewer of them, but they are more time-consuming.

Tip

Don't let yourself get stuck for too long on any one question. If you don't know, circle it and come back later. If you are waffling between two answers, go with your first instinct - it is usually correct.

Watch Out

If your exams are given with a "scantron" answer sheet (the kind requiring you to color in the circle of the correct response), be sure that the answers match up. Many students have found that when they "skip" a question, they forget to leave that line blank on the scantron. The result is that all their answers are recorded wrong.

Leave 5 minutes at the end of the exam for review. Go back over the test and check your answers. Make sure you filled in the correct dots or circled the answers you intended. Check over any calculations for simple math errors and the transposition of numbers. Make sure you have not left any question unanswered.

Preparing for Finals

Hopefully, you've been studying as you go. Studying for finals takes all semester. To be honest, you just can't cram for a final exam - it's not possible. The good news is, you have already taken tests on everything covered in your finals. You know this stuff already! To prepare for the final, you need to start at the beginning and review, one unit at a time.

Tip

Go over old tests and your notes from the term - check your memory. If there are holes, patch them. Take the time now to learn the things you let slide earlier in the semester. You can bet it will all be there on the final.

Chances are, you will have more than one final during finals week. You need to budget your time so you can adequately prepare for each one. Your best bet is to stick to one subject at a time during each study session. Jumping back and forth will confuse things.

As with regular studying, build in time for frequent breaks. You will retain more information for your finals in six 1-hour study sessions than two 3-hour sessions. Plus, it just feels less intimidating.

Finally, make sure you understand all the "big ticket items" - major concepts, theories, protocols, etc. Comprehensive finals will have more generalized questions than regular unit exams. You need a thorough understanding of the big picture. Once you have the major concepts down, you can then feel free to work in the details.

The Sun Will Rise Again

Post tenebras lux - after darkness, light.

So you bombed a test, huh? You're feeling pretty demoralized and downhearted about the whole thing. You may even be thinking of throwing in the towel. Don't!

Fact

First, let's have a reality check, okay?

◆ You are NOT the first person to ever fail an exam in nursing school. As a matter of fact, its pretty common - everyone tanks at least once.

◆ No one thinks any less of you - your teacher doesn't hate you or think you're a moron. Your classmates aren't snickering behind your back or wondering how you got into the program in the first place. These tests are HARD...everyone is very well aware of that fact.

◆ In the grand scheme of things, is it *really* the end of the world? It's one test. The sun will still rise tomorrow, whether you believe it will or not.

◆ One test does not a nurse make (or un-make). Just because you bombed one test does not mean you are destined to fail each succeeding one. You can definitely bounce back and find your stride again.

Pick yourself up, dust off and rededicate yourself to the program. Look at this as one of those "learning experiences" your mother told you about.

To understand what went wrong, evaluate why *you* think you performed poorly on this exam. Did you not put in enough study time? Were you having a hard time grasping the concepts? Did the questions throw you for a loop? Only you can answer these questions.

Tip

If adequate study time was the problem, look at ways to plan and prioritize better the next time around. If you were having a hard time with the concepts or material, check into your college's tutoring or student assistance programs. If you are not yet in a study group, join one! If the questions threw you for a loop - well, now you know. Next time, you will be better prepared for the kind of questions your instructor writes.

Don't Panic

The bottom line here is that you can get past this. Treat it as an isolated incident, learn from it and move on. You will still make a great nurse, and this one test does not in any way diminish your potential for excellence!

Research

Once upon a time, there was a nursing student named Nursey Lursey...

"Oh no, here we go again with the fables...you're going to tell us next that Nursey Lursey was a three-toed sloth maybe?"

No, of course not. Who ever heard of a three-toed sloth attending nursing school, silly? Now, on with the story...

Nursey Lursey was looking up some information on the internet for a school project, when she came upon a web page containing the following dire warning:
                The sky is falling - take cover!

Nursey Lursey panicked and ran into the basement, never to be heard from again.

...But the sky never did fall.

<ahem> The end.

"That's it? That was much shorter than the last one!"

The moral of the story?

Always evaluate your sources.

Poor Nursey Lursey - had she just taken the time to evaluate where this information was coming from, instead of taking it as solid truth, she would have learned the website was maintained by none other than Chicken Little - the scamp! Of course the sky wasn't falling - just because you see it in print, doesn't make it so.

The ocean of medical literature is vast and wide. For every one article proclaiming the absolute truth about something, there will be 10 more to discredit it. You can find any number of studies to support your ideas, but they don't necessarily amount to a hill of beans.

When it comes to research, whether you are looking something up online to help you understand a classroom concept, or researching a paper in the library, you have to evaluate your sources.

This section will briefly cover general research - the kinds of things you need to know when writing a paper on nursing theory or hunting for background information on diseases. It is not intended to provide information about the separate and wholly different discipline of nursing research - that we will leave up to your research class in *nursing* school.

Finding Information

So you need to write a paper on the ethics of nursing care for patients with cancer. Where can you find information? Your text books will have good information, but often you will need more than they will provide. You may have purchased some nursing reference books earlier on, but even then you may need more information. Where should you look?

The best place is, of course, your school's library. They will have more resources specific to your needs than the public library. If you haven't visited yours yet, pop over and take a tour. Talk with one of the librarians about how to find information in the most efficient manner - they will have tons of ideas to help make your research easier.

Don't Forget

Information evolves quickly in the medical field, so look for the most current material.

Another option is the internet. The world wide web is an amazing thing - billions of documents at your immediate disposal - and you don't even have to leave the comfort of your home. Type a few key words into the search engine and within seconds, a list of matches will be returned. The more specific your request, the better targeted this list will be, saving you time from wading through irrelevant websites. For example, if you are looking for articles about the ethics involved in the nursing care of cancer patients, you might run the following search:
Nursing ethics

In this case, you will be given a list of documents related to nursing ethics in general. You will find yourself digging for hours to find any article specific to the care of cancer patients. Truly, it will be like searching for a needle in a haystack.

If you enter the following search instead, you will have much better luck finding the information you seek:

Nursing ethics cancer care

Now the search engine will return a list of articles covering all four key words, and you should be able to find what you are looking for within the first two pages.

Don't Panic

Not exactly computer saavy? A little intimidated by the information super highway? Don't sweat it - it's not as difficult as it seems. As a matter of fact, once you've had a chance to get familiar with computers and the internet, you'll wonder why you waited so long! Check your college or university's course listings for introductory computer classes geared to beginners. These 1 to 3 credit hour courses allow you to learn about computers and the internet at your own pace.

bandidobooks.com

For more information on conducting internet searches, visit our website!

Evaluating Sources

You wouldn't get accounting advice from a shoe salesman or a zookeeper. Sure, they may have some helpful suggestions for you, but when your neck is on the chopping block with the IRS, you'll be wishing you had consulted an accountant, right? The same principle applies to medical and scientific information. You need to know where the information is coming from to decide just how valid it is. This concept is at the heart of evaluating your sources.

Things to ask yourself when considering evaluating information for accuracy:
- **Who is writing it?**
  Government agencies and educational institutions will have the most sound information. Private organizations and national groups often have good information, but it may be more subjective, based on their agenda. If an individual has created the work, what is this person's background in the industry and what are their credentials?
- **What are the references?**
  A sound article will have a list of quality resources and references used when developing the piece.
- **What is the motivation?**
  Sometimes an article that checks out on all other fronts has a problem with motive. Why are they writing this article? Is it political? Is it for fundraising purposes? Is it to solicit business? Make sure the motivation is in line with the information.

If in doubt, a final check is corroboration. If the same information appears in several reputable publications, it is most likely to be reliable. If you can only find one reference to a particular concept or theory, it may not be sound.

Drawing Conclusions

Care must be taken when drawing conclusions from a wide base of researched information. Make sure you think critically and only make logical statements based on fact. It is very easy to jump from point A to point C, but if you can't back it up with the intermediate step, point B, your credibility will be shot.

Case in point: Research shows that violent crimes skyrocket during the summer. Research also shows that ice cream sales increase significantly during the same period. A valid statement supported by research would be that violent crime and ice cream sales both increase during the summer. It would be a fallacy, however, to further conclude that the sale of ice cream has a direct impact on the occurrence of violent crime. The two are not related. It is hotter during the summer and people have shorter fuses, hence the increase in crime. Additionally, when it is hotter, people consume more ice cream, because it cools them off. While the two statistics share the common factor of heat, neither one is affected by, nor related to, the other.

Don't Forget

Research is an integral part of your nursing education (and practice!). The knowledge-base of the nursing profession is constantly changing and evolving; in order to provide the highest level of quality care, you need to continually update your knowledge of best practices and advances in treatment. Thus, when investigating clinical issues, use the tools at your disposal, evaluate your sources and, thinking critically, draw appropriate conclusions

The Joy of Clinicals

Clinicals are without a doubt the most important part of your nursing education. It is here that all your knowledge and skills are pulled together in real working situations. Your experiences in clinicals will improve your technique, expand your understanding of learned concepts, and build your confidence. This is where you *apply* what you have learned.

You will be assigned to a variety of clinical settings during your program. The idea is to expose you to as many areas of practice as possible prior to graduation. You may find yourself working in a hospital, an elementary school, a longterm care facility, a community health center and maybe even a few non-traditional settings, like an alternative healthcare facility or mobile clinic. You will have rotations in labor and delivery, pediatrics, geriatrics, the psychiatric unit, the operating room (O.R.) and medical-surgical units. You probably will be allowed to choose your own rotation during your senior year enabling you to get experience in an area matching your professional interest.

Clinicals are a wonderful experience and invaluable to your growth as a student of nursing. Enjoy them, and above all, *learn* from them - learn as much as you possibly can.

What Are They Like?

Most students are understandably nervous about clinicals. More than anything, it is the fear of the unknown. What are they like? What do I have to do? What if I make a mistake?

Let's look first at what they are like. The clinical experience is similar to having an actual job - you will be expected to show up on time, act professionally and dress appropriately for the assignment. You will be required to obey all the rules and regulations of the sponsoring facility, as well as those outlined by your school.

You are *not* going to be thrown into a life-or-death situation on your first day. As a matter of fact, you will spend your first clinical rotation perfecting the basics of care: making beds, giving baths, changing dressings, helping with transfers and taking vital signs.

You will also not be left alone. Your clinical instructor will be with you the whole way and you will probably have a student partner for those first clinical assignments. Also, you will most likely be assigned to work with a practicing nurse who will "precept" you and serve as a mentor and reference source. It is only after you have had significant clinical experience and have passed certain skills tests that you will slowly be given more autonomy. You have to earn the right, basically - and you will not be allowed to do anything you haven't already been trained to do.

As you progress through your rotations, you will be given more responsibility. You may manage two or three patients. You may be assigned to more difficult cases. Keep in mind though, that they will not give you anything you are not ready for. Hopefully this will ease your fears a little more.

There is one more thing you can count on - clinicals are exciting. You will be working with a diverse population of patients, right alongside nurses, physicians and other healthcare professionals. You will see and learn and do much more than you can imagine.

What Will I Be Expected to Do?

Experience is a hard teacher, because
she gives the test first, the lesson afterwards.

- Anonymous

During clinicals, you will be given a clear outline of what you can and cannot do. You will not be allowed to do things you have not practiced yet in labs...but you *will* be expected to do those things you have already learned.

Specifically:

- ✦ You will be expected to act as a functioning member of the care team.
- ✦ You will be required to treat patients holistically with respect for their individual needs.
- ✦ You will research you patient's condition ahead of each assignment and develop care plans for them.
- ✦ You will perform clinical assessments, make nursing diagnoses, outline interventions and provide patient-centered care.
- ✦ You will be required to follow universal precautions, document everything, act professionally and think on your feet.
- ✦ You will be expected to pitch in and help when needed.
- ✦ Finally, you will meet before and after each clinical day for a group conference to share experiences with (and get feedback from) your instructor and peers.

Watch Out

Normally, in a hospital, there are sick people - duh! The point is that nurses have to not only care for and protect their patients, but also themselves! Most likely, early in your clinicals you will be exposed to a wide variety of communicable diseases (stuff you can catch!) as well as to potentially violent patients (i.e., mentally ill patients on any unit/floor, or in a psychiatric unit). Practice universal precautions and be aware of unit specific or patient specific guidelines and protocols. Above all, practice common sense and *wash your hands!*

There is an important concept of *progression* in clinicals - each new skill builds on the last. As you master one skill, you move on to the next. It is important that you keep moving forward in your clinicals, continually adding to your "nursing tool box" of skills and knowledge.

What do your instructors expect of you during your assignment? Read on...

Point of View: A Clinical Instructor

As a clinical instructor, what do you expect from students?
The things I expect from my students are:
✦ Ethical and critical thinking when making decisions about client care.
✦ Valuing client needs.
✦ Application of previous clinical concepts and skills to present clinical.
✦ Collegial sharing of experiences in pre/post conferences.

In your opinion, what is most important?
✦ Progression within the clinical.
✦ Frequent communication with the instructor, via documentation or verbal communication.
✦ Holistic assessment and nursing diagnosis of client.

What are you looking for when evaluating students?
✦ Demonstration of professionalism.
✦ Evidence of client leadership and management of care.
✦ Self-direction and initiative in providing for their learning needs.
✦ Organization of client care.
✦ Client assessment and teaching.

- Patricia Bennett, RN, MSN
Assistant Professor, Molloy College

Helpful Advice

Practice good etiquette and common courtesy during each of your clinical rotations:
✦ Introduce yourself to the nurses on duty.
✦ Ask if you can help out in any way.
✦ Respect their territory and their time.
✦ Always be polite.

Keep the lines of communication wide open with your instructor. If you are unsure about *anything* - ask. They would rather walk you through it now, than try to clean up a disaster after the fact. Keep them informed.

Don't try to cover up mistakes. This is a learning environment - no one just waltzes out of class performing every procedure and protocol to perfection. Take responsibility for your actions and be honest.

Don't be afraid to try. When presented with a new learning opportunity or challenge, take it! It's going to come up again later in your career, you can count on it. Better to try it now, under the protective wing of your instructor.

Getting the Experience You Need

I hear and I forget. I see and I remember. I do and I understand.

- Confucius

In keeping with the concept of progression, you need to seek out experiences that will add to your growth and development as a nurse. If you would like a specific assignment, ask for it! If you see a nurse performing a procedure you haven't done yet, ask to watch, or if appropriate, to assist. If there is a certain technique you want a more practice with, ask your instructor to keep an eye out for extra learning opportunities.

Don't Forget

Remember, it won't be too long before you are out in the real world working as a nurse. Be proactive - take the initiative to get the experiences you need. These are *your* clinicals.

Care Plans

"We keep hearing about these care plan things - what the heck are they?"

A care plan is a written plan of action tailored specifically to the needs of your client. It takes into account the nursing diagnosis (see below), current patient condition, historical data and any other pertinent information related to your client's well-being. In writing the care plan, you will develop goals and expected outcomes for your patient, outlining what nursing interventions you will use to facilitate this process and how you will evaluate them.

In a nutshell, it says, "Patient X has problem Y. Here's what we're gonna do to help him get better." Of course, it's much more than that, but that's the main idea.

Students spend *a lot* of time writing care plans, and really, this is a good thing. Care plans guide you to most effectively meeting the needs of your patient. They help you set priorities for care and keep you focused on the holistic needs of the patient as a person, not just a body with a disease.

Nursing Diagnoses

A nursing diagnosis is a statement of an actual or potential health problem that can be resolved through the assistance of nursing interventions. This is the starting off point for creating a comprehensive care plan. In order to treat a patient, you have to identify what the problem areas are.

Nursing diagnoses are not to be confused with medical diagnoses of conditions. A medical diagnosis is "patient has pneumonia." A possible nursing diagnosis for this same patient could be "patient has ineffective airway clearance." See the difference? A nursing diagnosis evaluates the patient and the problems they are experiencing as a result of, or in response to, the medically diagnosed condition or disease.

A licensed professional nurse has the authority and autonomy to formulate and to treat nursing diagnoses. Physicians, on the other hand, treat medical diagnoses. In our example, the physician might prescribe an antibiotic to combat the pneumonia, while the nurse might instruct the patient in breathing/coughing exercises or encourage fluids to facilitate efficient breathing.

In practice, the clinical setting is a collaborative process including the efforts of many healthcare professionals. Nurses practice in this environment through actions, some independent (like the formulation of a care plan) and some dependent (like following the physician's order to administer the antibiotic).

Don't Panic

Do not be intimidated by the terminology of "diagnosis" or the process of "care plans." These, like others systems in use (i.e., *Nursing Intervention Classification* -NIC and *Nursing Outcome Classification* -NOC) are tools to help you organize, deliver and evaluate your care and practice. See them as your allies, not as stumbling blocks.

Holistic Care

Holistic (or wholistic) care is at the heart of the nursing profession. Nurses are taught to treat the person as a whole and to look at things from as many angles as possible. The object is to get the most accurate and complete perspective of the true needs of the patient. Areas to evaluate with a holistic approach include the physical, mental, emotional and spiritual needs of each person as an individual. Familial support, environment, nutrition and stress are also factors considered when evaluating a patient's ability to regain and maintain health.

Cultural Issues in Nursing

When love and skill work together, expect a masterpiece.

- John Ruskin

Providing holistic care also means being sensitive to and respectful of cultural differences. What is best for you, based on your beliefs and background, may not be appropriate or make any sense for a patient of a different cultural heritage. As a nurse (and nursing student), you need to try to understand these differences so you can more effectively care for your patient. Above all, you must be willing to give excellent, objective care despite differences in belief or practice, even if said beliefs are in direct conflict with your own. A nurse refrains from being judgmental; rather a nurse recognizes the intrinsic value and worth of each person individually.

Multicultural Care

Nursing is a noble profession, a calling, and a physical and emotional challenge with a humanly fulfilling moral mission. As a nurse, you will encounter patients in their most vulnerable moments, sharing an intimacy that is only found in few other human relationships.

In a world that is rapidly becoming multicultural, the nurse must develop sensitivity to his/her own fundamental values regarding health and illness. This, in turn, will set up the framework to give you the courage to accept the existence of differing values and make you think about the care of people from diverse cultures.

It is not easy to alter attitudes and beliefs, or stereotypes and prejudices, but it is imperative that nurses have a sound understanding and knowledge related to the nursing care of patients who value their cultural heritage and life ways. Do not make assumptions and do respect differences. Recognize that other people's views are just as valid as your own.

- Victor M. Fernandez, RN, CEN, BSN
- Kathleen M. Fernandez, RN-C, BSN
Transcultural Nursing: Basic Concepts and Case Studies

bandidobooks.com

Interpersonal Skills

You communication skills are extremely important during clinicals. You must be able to interact well with your instructor, the staff on duty and your patients.

Here are some rules of the road to keep in mind:

- ✦ Use good eye contact, especially with patients.
- ✦ ALWAYS keep in mind your patient's dignity.
- ✦ Watch your body language - your mouth may be saying one thing while your body is saying something completely different.
- ✦ Similarly, watch the tone of your voice. Slight variations in tone can change the perceived meaning behind your words.
- ✦ Listen - really listen. When someone is talking to you, stop what you are doing and give them your full attention.
- ✦ Never contradict your instructor, the nurses on duty or other healthcare professionals in front of a patient. Wait until you are able to discuss it with them in private.
- ✦ Never gossip about your patients, or anyone else for that matter - its unprofessional and reflects poorly on you.
- ✦ Don't whine, complain or gripe around patients - it's not their fault you are there. Besides, how would that make you feel if you were the patient? Same thing applies to comments made around facility staff.
- ✦ Be considerate, respectful, friendly and professional
  Above all, remember to smile...a friendly smile and a positive attitude will take you far.

Watch Out

Respecting patient confidentiality is not just good etiquette - it's an ethical cornerstone of the profession <u>and</u> it's the law. It is *never* appropriate to discuss a patient's medical condition or personal circumstances outside of the confines of nursing practice. Sharing private information, even with a family member, is a big no-no. At the very least, a lax attitude towards patient confidentiality can get you kicked out of school. From an ethical perspective, it's a breach of the sacred trust between healthcare providers and those they serve. From a legal perspective, you could be held personally liable for divulging confidential information.

Maximize Your Educational Experience

Remember our friend, the platypus? She realized that learning to be a nurse went beyond books and clinicals. She was a student of humanity. She looked at everything as an opportunity to experience greater personal and professional growth. She looked beyond herself to see the world around her, and actively sought ways to contribute.

Don't spend all your time in school buried in books. Look up from time to time - there is so much going on around you. You have the chance to get involved in things, to make a difference in the profession and the world. It's never too early to get started, nor is it ever too late.

Get Involved

Here is the test to find whether your mission on Earth is finished:
If you're alive, it isn't.

- Richard Bach

Consider joining extracurricular clubs and associations. Student organizations offer you the opportunity to hold offices, join committees and become politically active. They are also a great source of fellowship and mentoring.

One organization you will want to be a part of is the National Student Nurses' Association (NSNA). The NSNA is a pre-professional organization specifically for nursing students. It has local chapters at most accredited schools of nursing, as well as state and national offices.

As with professional associations, the NSNA unifies and represents its constituents. Members are able to network with peers, make valuable professional contacts and keep up-to-date on the latest legislation and happenings in the world of nursing. Additionally, participation at the local chapter level offers great opportunities for leadership and mentoring.

Other benefits of joining the NSNA include scholarships, low-cost insurance and student loan programs, an online career center and access to a variety of NSNA publications. For more information, check into your school's chapter, or contact:

National Student Nurses' Association
555 W. 57th Street
New York, NY 10019
(212) 581-2211

bandidobooks.com

Check out our website for more ways to get involved!

Keep in mind that the foundation and continued growth of the nursing profession is vitally dependent on the leadership and participation of its members. Your participation counts - get involved!

Give Something Back

To the world, you might be one person,
But to one person, you might be the world.

- Anonymous

Consider volunteer work in the healthcare field. It allows you the chance to further hone your skills and gain valuable experience, while giving something back to your community and neighbors. The personal rewards of volunteering cannot be measured.

The Red Cross is one such notable organization offering a variety of volunteer opportunities specifically for nursing students. Student nurses can teach public safety courses such as First Aid, CPR, and swimming. They can participate in health fairs, immunization and blood drives, public health screenings and disaster relief. They can serve as active members on planning committees or can even become part of the public speaking team. There are plenty of options available to suit your personal schedule and interests.

A special form of recognition is given to nursing students who volunteer for this agency: the *American Red Cross Nursing Pin*. After only 10 hours of service to the Red Cross, you will receive a silver and blue pin inscribed with the words, "Student Nurse...Answering Humanity's Call."

For more information, call your local American Red Cross office, or contact the Office of the Chief Nurse at their national headquarters - (202) 639-3145.

Check out our website for more volunteer opportunities.

bandidobooks.com

Take Care of Yourself

How do you get out of debt? Pay yourself first. Interesting, isn't it? One would think the way to get out of debt would be to pay your bills or get a second job. But no, the first step to getting out of debt is saving money.

If you always spend your entire paycheck paying down bills, you will never have a savings cushion for emergencies. And there are always emergencies; that's just life. Where does the money come from if you don't have savings? You have to borrow more. So, when you don't pay yourself first before paying others, you are, in effect, digging your hole deeper. The bills will still be there either way - it's your choice.

The same thing applies to your life. If you spend every ounce of your energy on school, family and work responsibilities, you will be exhausted. Without making time for yourself to recharge - banking a reserve of energy to draw on - you will be running on borrowed time. You will continue to fall farther and farther behind until finally, you feel so overwhelmed you can no longer act. Pay yourself first. There will always be a list of Very-Important-Things you have to get done - it's your choice.

Balancing School, Work and Family

The sun will set without your assistance.

- The Talmud

Love that quote - the sun will set without your assistance. Apparently, these folks have drastically underestimated our pivotal place in the grand scheme of things. And who was that other guy...Gallileo? Yeah, that's him. He had some crazy notion that the universe does not revolve around us. Has anyone evaluated his sources on this yet? It sounds fishy. Obviously the world would cease to function if we did not micromanage every aspect of our lives, right?

Wrong! The world truly does NOT rest on your shoulders - and, if you recall from your history lessons, it managed quite nicely without your intervention for, oh...several billion years, but who's counting? It wouldn't hurt you to let go of some of that control just a little bit.

Before you can interject here, let's just list off the "Yes, but's" currently floating through your mind:

YES, BUT:

My employer is depending on me to handle (insert Very Important Task here), and if I don't do it, it won't be done right. If it's not done right, business will falter, the company will go into bankruptcy, the stock market will crash and the country will be plunged into a depression the likes of which have not been seen for over 80 years.

***

If I miss out on one single moment of my children's lives, they will be scarred for life and will never forgive my moment of selfish indulgence. Twenty years from now, their faces will be plastered on the FBI's Most Wanted List, and as the subjects of an international manhunt, they will be charged with money laundering, spearheading the world's largest drug cartel and littering on public sidewalks. As the press closes in on them after their capture, they will be quoted as saying, "I did it because I was unloved as a child - my mother never made time for me!"

***

If I do not keep the house immaculate myself, nothing will ever get done. Laundry will pile to the ceiling, the grass will stand unmowed until the house is hidden from view, small woodland creatures will make their homes in the cupboards and rafters, and the dust bunnies will evolve into intelligent life. Our neighbors will be ashamed to walk on the same side of the street as us, the city planning commission will condemn our house and we will all be out on the streets - homeless, I say - HOMELESS!

Should we continue? Thought not. You know none of this is logical or realistic, but it sure feels like it sometimes, right? How incredibly heavy is that burden you are current-ly carrying around with you? No wonder you're worn out! Never fear, help is on the way.

The first thing you need to do is let go. Set some of that stuff down. Does it *really* matter if the laundry only gets done once a week, or if you ask your children to help with the dishes? Is there no way you can delegate some of your responsibilities at work? Delegation is the hallmark of a good manager, you know...

Tip

Try these helpful hints on for size:

<u>At Home</u>

✦ Get your family involved - encourage their support and ask for their suggestions.

✦ Divide up household responsibilities - even little ones can put their own laundry away or help dust.

✦ Lower your standards - even just a little will help.

✦ Set aside one day of the week for "family time" - stick to it - no schoolwork whatsoever. Your family will be more willing to accommodate your needs during the week if they feel like they are also a priority.

<u>At Work</u>

✦ If possible, cut back to part-time or request flexible scheduling

✦ Communicate frequently with your supervisors - let them know what's going on and what may come up

✦ Delegate, delegate, delegate - pass along whatever you can

✦ Don't be afraid to say "no." You do not have to accept every assignment offered to you.

When all else fails, ask yourself, "How important is this item?" Is it so important you would be willing to lose your left leg to get it done? No? Your finger? No? Your little toe? You never really use it you know. No? Well then, maybe in the grand scheme of things, it's really not that important after all...maybe it can be adjusted. Don't believe this line of reasoning works? Ask yourself the question again, this time as follows: "How important is it that I save my child from a burning house?" Now you see the difference.

Making Time for Yourself

Remember our talk about the energy reserve bank you need to be adding to on a regular basis? We weren't kidding - it is important. YOU are important. You won't be able to do anything well if you aren't taking care of yourself. Don't neglect your own needs.

Think of some creative ways to make a deposit into that savings account - making time for yourself doesn't have to cost money - it just has to make you feel good again. Here are some favorites I like:

✦ Slip away to the bookstore for a few hours. Use those big comfy chairs they have throughout the store to curl up and read a good book.

✦ Talk a walk - the exercise will rejuvenate your body while the sunshine rejuvenates your spirits.

- ✦ Indulge in a bubble bath, and pull out all the stops - scented candles, bath oils, music - what were you saving them for anyway?
- ✦ Pamper yourself a bit - get your hair done, go shopping, eat a decadent dessert.
- ✦ Have a night out on the town with your friends.
- ✦ Focus on the arts - visit the art gallery or history museum, take in a play or musical, paint a picture, draw or write. Sing!
- ✦ Take up yoga. Or dance. Or tennis. Or golf. Try something new.
- ✦ Sleep in - just once - until 11:00 a.m. Have breakfast in bed. Don't get dressed all day.
- ✦ Rent a funny movie. Order take-out. Stay up past your bedtime.
- ✦ Call up an old friend you haven't talked to in years.
- ✦ Find out how many licks it takes to get to the center of a Tootsie Pop (and when you do, let me know!)

Adjust Your Attitude

Sometimes, a simple attitude adjustment can do wonders for your outlook and give you a much-needed boost. The way you look at things is a choice. All events are neutral - it is only our interpretation of them that attaches a negative or positive connotation. You may not have control over some of the things that happen in your life, but you DO have control over how you choose to view them.

A Native American elder once described his own inner struggles in this manner:

"Inside of me there are two dogs.
One of the dogs is mean and evil.
The other dog is good.
The mean dog fights the good dog all the time."

When asked which dog wins, he reflected for a moment and replied,

"The one I feed the most."

Be Assertive

How you choose to handle yourself also affects you state of mind. Being assertive allows you to communicate your feelings in a direct and honest manner.

What exactly is being assertive? According to Merriam-Webster's dictionary, being assertive means "to state positively, to affirm." It means expressing what you want to say in a manner that respects your rights and needs, as well as the rights and needs of others.

This is not to be confused with being aggressive, wherein we put our own rights and needs above those of everyone else. It also differs from being non-assertive, where more value is placed on others' needs than our own.

Next time you are confronted with an uncomfortable or emotionally-charged situation, try using the following techniques to express yourself assertively - see if it doesn't make an enormous difference!

+ **"When this happened, I felt..."**

   Instead of saying, "You obviously don't care about your students!" try, "When you didn't allow me to explain why I had a hard time with that procedure, I felt minimized."

+ **Focus on "I" instead of "you." Take ownership.**

   Instead of saying, "You didn't give me a second chance!" try, "I would like the opportunity to try this again so I can improve my technique."

+ **Be specific.**

   Instead of saying, "This assignment is too hard!" try, "The instructions for completing this exercise are confusing to me. Can we go over it again briefly?"

+ **Use the facts.**

   Instead of saying, "You never do your share of the work!" try, "You didn't complete your section of the study guide in time for our group meeting. That is the fourth time this month."

+ **Show cause and effect.**

   Instead of saying, "You are completely insensitive!" try, "I get frustrated when you show up late for our study group. We have to stop our work to catch you up, then start at the beginning again."

+ **Suggest an equitable resolution.**

   Instead of saying, "You talk too fast during your lectures - how is anyone supposed to keep up?!" try, "Your class moves pretty quickly and covers a lot of important material. Would it be alright to record your lectures?"

Motivation

The brook would lose its song if you removed the stones.

- Anonymous

Sometimes when we overdo it, we get burned out - we lose our motivation. In nursing school, you are under tremendous pressure. The payoff is not immediate, so the reward for your struggles can appear to be perpetually out of reach. There may come a time when you feel so stressed out, you are ready to give up.

Well folks, desperate times call for desperate measures. At crossroads like this, take a time out. Focus on why you are doing this - remember your reasons for applying to nursing school in the first place. Find one thing - just one thing to hold on to, to keep you going until your motivation returns. How about these for starters:

"Mommy, I am so proud of you."

"I was really scared before the operation - thank you for sitting with me and making me feel less alone."

"You're going to make a great nurse someday - keep up the good work!"

Think about what nursing means to you - remember what it was all about at the beginning - making a difference in people's lives. Being a healer. Proving to yourself that you could do it.

Look forward - keep your focus on graduation day, the pinning ceremony, getting your license, finding your dream job, saving lives.

Your heart is in nursing - don't lose sight of that. It's hard work now, but it is so very worth it.

Keep Your Eye on the Prize

If I had but one piece of advice for students entering nursing school, it would be this: Keep your eye on the prize! The demands on your time and your talents are extreme. Just keep in mind that it doesn't last forever, and the prize will be worth it. Study hard, relax when you can, budget your time and reward yourself often!

- Louise Komorek, BSN student
Southern Illinois University

Graduation Day

Finally, your day to shine has arrived. All those years of hard work and sacrifice have paid off. You are about to graduate from nursing school and embark upon the career of a lifetime. Believe it - you did it!

There will be celebration parties, special brunches, recruiting functions and awards ceremonies. Your social calendar, which has spent the last two years collecting dust, will now be full to the brim. It will all culminate with the beloved pinning ceremony and your graduation. Be proud of yourself and stand tall in the spotlight, for you have earned the right to be there. Above all, enjoy this time and savor every minute. You will never forget these last few weeks.

The Pinning Ceremony

The Pinning Ceremony is a time-honored nursing school tradition. Often more personally meaningful than the graduation ceremony, it signifies your official initiation into the brotherhood and sisterhood of nurses. The ceremony is rich in symbolism and deeply moving. It is a rite of passage dating back to the late 19th century.

The history of the Pinning Ceremony is quite interesting, and can be traced all the way back to the Crusades in the 12th century. During this time, the Knights of the Order of the Hospital of St. John the Baptist tended to injured and infirm Crusaders. When new monks were initiated into the order, they vowed to serve these sick soldiers. In a special ceremony, each new monk was presented with a Maltese cross - the first badges given to those who nurse.

The modern ceremony dates back to the 1860's when Florence Nightingale was awarded the Red Cross of St. George in recognition of her tireless service to the injured in the Crimean War. Wanting to share this honor somehow with the brightest graduates of her nursing school, she presented them each with a medal of excellence.

The idea caught on and other schools began honoring graduates with special badges or pins. By 1916, the practice of pinning new graduates was standard throughout the U.S.

The ceremony itself is beautiful and quite emotional. New nurses recite the Nightingale Pledge and light a candle to guide them on their path. They are then each pinned with the nursing pin, a symbol of their pledge to work for the betterment of humankind and their membership in the profession. Schools often also add their own traditions into the ceremony as they welcome new nurses to the fold. The Pinning Ceremony is elegant in its simplicity, but for graduating students, its is a profoundly meaningful life event.

What's Next?

Don't get too comfortable yet, graduate nurse. You still have to take the NCLEX licensing exam before you will be an official RN or LPN. In the interim, you will be eligible for a temporary permit to practice as a graduate nurse. Typically good for 90 days (it can vary by state), this will allow you to find employment while waiting on the your new license. There's lots to be done still, so take a deep breath and get ready to move on to the next phase - *transitioning to the real world of nursing.*

Part III

Now that you've graduated, you are a few short steps away from your career as a nursing professional. This section will help you soar over the final hurdles, from passing the NCLEX licensing exam to finding your dream job to coping during the first six months on the job.

The Dreaded NCLEX

NCLEX - dare I even say the word aloud? It's the final hurdle to becoming a licensed nurse. There is such an aura of mystery about it - from its unique method of selecting questions, to how it defines your level of knowledge - that most folks are terrified. And with so much riding on the final result, it puts enormous pressure on new grads.

Some will tell you there is no way to prepare for the NCLEX - they will say you can't study for it, you can't even begin to fathom how hard it is, and you can't prepare yourself for how unnerved it will leave you.

Relax - it is *not* that bad. Difficult? Sure - as it should be. Impossible? No. In the year 2000, 80% of NCLEX-RN takers (graduates of RN programs) passed the exam on the first try. That means 4 out of 5 people will pass on their first attempt - pretty good odds, don't you think? The pass rate is even higher for the NCLEX-PN (for graduates of LPN programs) at 84%.

As for preparation, there are lots of resources available to help you prepare for the NCLEX - review courses, books, practice exams - and many nursing instructors offer private tutoring. There *are* things you can do to get ready for this big test, if you choose to take advantage of them.

The surprise factor can be eliminated simply by learning about the exam itself. Finding out as much as you can about the test *ahead* of time will leave you feeling more centered and less apprehensive, decreasing the likelihood of the test throwing you for a loop. In this section, we'll take a close look at the NCLEX and what you can expect to encounter at the testing center.

The most important thing to remember is that you've already invested significant time studying for this exam, whether you realize it or not. From day one of your nursing classes, you have been steadily gathering a broad base of knowledge to draw on, while fine-tuning your critical thinking skills. Everything you have learned on your nursing school journey will pull together for you now during this last comprehensive test. You know more than you think you do. If you have made it this far, you are ready for the NCLEX.

What is it and How Does it Work?

Fact

NCLEX stands for National Council Licensure Examination. It is a standardized, national exam designed to measure and evaluate competencies in nursing. All graduates of nursing programs are required to successfully pass this exam in order to obtain their professional license. Without this license, you cannot legally practice nursing.

The National Council of State Boards of Nursing develops the NCLEX exam. These are the folks who oversee professional licensing, nursing policy and professional regulation. Their Board of Directors determine the passing standard, or minimum level of competency, for the exam.

Test questions are written by a panel of qualified nurse volunteers with experience in a wide range of clinical settings and nursing practice areas. Thousands of questions have been written, evaluated and approved for use in the test data bank. The aim is to provide a diverse collection of questions applicable to entry-level nursing scope of practice and activities. In simpler terms, these questions cover what new nurses need to know to effectively and safely provide nursing care.

The NCLEX is probably unlike any other test you have taken. Its methodology is unique:

+ Pass/fail is not determined by how many questions you get right; the test is designed so that *all* candidates get 50% right, 50% wrong.
+ Each candidate gets a different set of questions, since they are drawn from a test bank.
+ Everyone has a different *number* of questions - some may have as few as 75, while others may have 265. Incidentally, the number of questions has little relevance to whether or not you passed.
+ The better you do, the harder your questions get. If you get the first one correct, the second one will be harder.
+ You cannot skip questions, nor can you go back and change any answers - you get one shot at each question.

Nervous yet? Confused? Let's look at how *exactly* the NCLEX works.

The NCLEX uses what is called *computerized adaptive testing* (CAT). This method of test delivery employs a computer program that adapts the test to each individual, based on their answers. Each time you answer a question, two things happen:
1. The computer uses measurement theory to estimate your competency level. It looks at all previously answered questions to make this assessment.
2. Based on its findings, it selects another question for you to further evaluate your level of knowledge.
The program is designed to locate your exact level of competence. By giving you questions of varying difficulty covering a range of predefined areas, it is able to close in on how much you know.

Let's say the first question given to you is really difficult and you get it wrong. The computer says to itself, "Okay, that was too hard. Let's try something a little easier." It picks a question for you that is not quite so hard, and you get it right. "Aha!" says the computer, "This student's level of knowledge falls somewhere in between the really difficult question and the easier question." It continues to give you harder or easier questions based on your answers, and evaluates your performance after each one to find your exact level of knowledge. The exam will continue until an accurate pass/fail decision can be made. Everyone will get exactly half of the questions right, and half of them wrong.

During this process, the computer is also selecting questions for you that cover a wide range of practice areas. You cannot be evaluated on just a few of these predefined *test plan areas*, as they are called - your exam must include a minimum percentage of questions from each area to produce a valid profile of your level of competence. This makes it fair for everyone by ensuring that you don't end up with say 75 questions on infection control. You will be evaluated on all of the test plan areas during the exam. The are currently four test plan areas (main categories):

- ◆ Safe and effective care environment.
- ◆ Health promotion and maintenance.
- ◆ Psychosocial integrity.
- ◆ Physiological integrity.

Each of these main categories will include a combination of questions from the following ten subcategories:

- ◆ Management of care.
- ◆ Safety and infection control.
- ◆ Growth and development.
- ◆ Prevention and early detection of disease.
- ◆ Coping/adaptation.
- ◆ Psychosocial adaptation.
- ◆ Basic care and comfort.
- ◆ Pharmacological and parenteral therapies.
- ◆ Reduction of risk potential.
- ◆ Physiological adaptation.

Questions on the NCLEX are *integrated*. This means a single question could test on more than one category or subcategory. It makes sense - in a real nursing situation, you would not have a patient present with only one issue to evaluate. You need to be able to think critically and draw on information from many different areas when assessing patients and planning care. The exam reflects this.

The questions are presented in multiple choice format, with 4 possible answer choices per question. You can only answer each question once - you cannot go back and change an answer, nor can you skip questions. This is because of the way the CAT system is designed.

You will have up to 5 hours to complete the exam. There is a mandatory 10-minute break after the first two hours, and you can take an additional break (optional) one and a half hours after that. The test will shut off at 5 hours whether it has finished assessing your level of competence or not.

There is no maximum time limit for an individual question, so you can take as much time as you need. The minimum number of questions you can receive is 75, and the maximum is 205 for the NCLEX-PN, 265 for the NCLEX-RN. Most people fall somewhere in between.

Don't Panic

The exam is conducted, obviously, via computer. You do NOT have to know how to use a computer. If you can point and click with a mouse, or use the space bar and "enter" key, you will be fine. All the other keys are disconnected, so you can't botch things up. You will also be given instructions ahead of time, a brief computer/mouse tutorial and a practice exercise so you can get a feel for things.

The NCLEX exams are now administered at Sylvan Learning Centers across the country. In the pre-CAT era, tests were taken with paper and pencil, and were only scheduled twice a year. Now, you can schedule the date and time of your exam individually to fit your particular needs.

You will not be allowed to take anything into the exam with you other than required identification - purses, books, etc. will need to be left outside of the testing area. You will sit in an individual computer cubicle during your exam and it's very quiet in there - don't let that unnerve you.

When the exam is over, the computer will shut off. You will not be given any indication of how you did - it will just end. Don't let this rattle you either, and don't worry if you only got so many questions or if the last question was really easy or hard. None of these are indicative of your performance.

NCLEX Myths

The anxiety factor tied to the NCLEX lends itself to widespread rumors about how the exam works and speculation about changes in the testing protocol. The National Council of State Boards of Nursing (NCSBN) is the only reliable source of information to debunk these myths.

Current myths addressed by the NCSBN include the following:

MYTH: *Beginning April 1, 2001, the NCLEX will change from multiple choice questions to fill-in-the-blank and essay questions.*
REALITY: Untrue. The NCSBN has been testing innovative new test formats, but -as of printing, none of these have yet been approved for use in the national NCLEX exam.

MYTH: *Some NCLEX questions require answers outside of the scope of practice for nurses.*
REALITY: Untrue. ALL test questions have been reviewed and approved by the Exam Committee and are within the scope of nursing practice.

MYTH: *Some candidates are randomly selected to receive the maximum number of questions regardless of performance on the exam.*
REALITY: Untrue. No candidate receives a pre-selected number of questions. The CAT system gives questions until it has accurately determined the candidate's level of competence, and then the test stops.

MYTH: *If you only get 75 questions on the exam and the last one was easy, you didn't pass.*
REALITY: Untrue. The number of questions is not indicative of passing or failing - it just means the computer needed fewer or more questions to evaluate your competence. Additionally, the exam is designed to give you a proportional number of questions from the predefined test plan areas. The last question is not indicative of your competence level.

MYTH: *NCLEX questions with pictures do not count in your score - they are new questions being tested by the review committee.*
REALITY: Untrue. Questions with graphics count. Moreover, they are not new to the test - they have been in use for many years.

MYTH: *Some states require a higher passing standard for licensure than others.*
REALITY: Untrue. All state boards of nursing accept the national council's passing standard to determine eligibility for licensure.

MYTH: *Only a certain percentage of candidates are allowed to pass each year.*
REALITY: Untrue. There is no fixed passing percentage or maximum number of candidates allowed to pass each year. Any candidate who, by assessment of their performance on the exam, is determined to meet or exceed the standard required of entry-level competency will pass.

MYTH: *You will receive 15 "test" questions on the exam - questions that are new and do not count towards your pass/fail percentage.*
REALITY: True. You will receive 15 questions that are currently being evaluated and are not yet part of the NCLEX exam. Your answers to these questions do not count towards your pass/fail percentage. However, you have no way of knowing which questions these are - they are not identified as "test" questions.

MYTH: *Starting April 1, 2001, NCLEX takers will be allowed to use the computer's calculator during the exam.*
REALITY: True. The NCSBN approved and implemented the use of an onscreen, drop-down calculator beginning in the spring of 2001. Candidates are allowed to use this tool during the exam.

Ask

For more information on the NCLEX, contact:
National Council of State Boards of Nursing
676 N. St. Clair Street, Suite 550
Chicago, IL 60611-2921
(312) 787-6555
e-mail: nclexinfo@ncsbn.org

Getting Ready for the Big Day

Trust yourself. You know more than you think you do.
- Benjamin Spock, M.D.

Is there really anything you can do to prepare for the NCLEX? Of course there is. As a matter of fact, there are lots of resources out there for you to use:
✦ **Review courses**
Check with your college or university to see if they offer a review class, or if they can refer you to other local resources.
✦ **Exam prep books and interactive CDs**
You can purchase these at your local bookstore, or check them out of your school's library.

bandidobooks.com

✦ **Practice Exams**
There are many sites on the internet that offer practice exams for a nominal charge. A limited number of sites offer free practice tests - but you have to search a little harder to find them. Visit our web site for a list of free practice exams online.
✦ **Tutors**
Many nursing instructors offer NCLEX tutoring. Ask around at your school to see which instructors accept students for tutoring.

Tip

Also, don't underestimate the power of your study group - after all, you got through nursing school together. It makes sense to band together one more time to prepare for the NCLEX. Bonus points: it's *free*. Pool your resources and work together.

When you are studying for the NCLEX, go slow and steady. Work on review for one to two hours a day, more if you feel like it - but don't overdo it. Consistency is more effective than cramming round the clock until you burn out.

Focus on the test plan areas - quiz yourself and study up on things that have faded from memory or about which you feel uncertain. Remember that the exam will give you integrated questions - you will have to apply knowledge from several areas to evaluate the question and come to an appropriate answer.

Finally, don't stay up studying until 3:00 a.m. the night before your exam. You will be a mess the next day if you do. There is nothing you can learn in the last 24 hours that will make the difference between passing and failing. Rest easy knowing you have done a thorough job preparing and get a good night's sleep. Eat breakfast in the morning. You will be able to concentrate better during the exam if you feel fresh, and a healthy breakfast will give you the energy you need to stay focused.

Waiting for the Results

The hardest part about the NCLEX is not taking it - it's waiting for the results. Waiting for the pass/fail notice can take anywhere from 5 days to a full month. The average wait is 2 weeks, but it feels like forever.

I have received countless inquiries about a magical web site that will give you your NCLEX results right away. Unfortunately this is just another myth - there is no web site where you can look up online whether you passed or failed.

There IS, however, a magical 900 number...it will cost you $7.95, but for some, the peace of mind is worth the fee. NCLEX Exam Results By Phone is a service that will give you the unofficial results of your exam. Candidates must wait three business days after taking the exam to call for the results, and a flat charge of $7.95 will appear on their phone bill, regardless of the length of the call. Be aware that only 17 states currently participate in this service. They are:

Arizona, Colorado, Delaware, Georgia, Iowa, Kansas,
Maine, Minnesota, Missouri, North Dakota, Nebraska,
New Jersey, New York, South Dakota, Utah,
West Virginia (PN only), Wisconsin

If you live in one of those states, you can use this service by calling 1-900-225-6000. Remember, you need to wait three business days after the exam to get the unofficial results.

For those who do not live in one of the states mentioned above, check to see if your state board of nursing has a automated license verification line. If so, you can call to see if you're listed as a licensed nurse (they may have the information in their system before you get your letter). Keep in mind that this will only let you know that you passed. If you cannot verify your license, it could mean you didn't pass, or just as easily, that they haven't received the information yet.

Don't call your state board of nursing's regular number asking for your NCLEX results -official results cannot be released over the phone. You may just have to wait to get the results the old-fashioned way - through the mail. Hang in there and try to find something to occupy your time - the letter will arrive before you know it.

If You Don't Pass...

It's not the end of the world if you don't pass the exam, nor does it automatically mean you are not fit for the nursing profession. You can take the test again.

If you did not pass the NCLEX, you will receive a Diagnostic Profile in the mail from your state board of nursing. This is a tool you can use to determine how close you were to passing and what areas you need to work on.

The Diagnostic Profile includes an overall performance assessment that will show you exactly how you scored, relative to the passing mark. Additionally, it will include a break-out of your performance in each of the test plan areas, highlighting your strengths and weaknesses. It will tell you which areas you need to improve in, and how much improvement will be necessary to pass. Using the Diagnostic Profile will help you decide which areas to focus on as you prepare to take the NCLEX again.

The NCSBN requires a minimum waiting period of 91 days before you can take the test again. Some state boards of nursing have additional requirements for retests - check with your home state's board. Contact information for all the boards are included in the Resources section of this book.

The most important thing is to not let one failure destroy your confidence or hopes of becoming a nurse. It happens...but it is not the end of the line. Many excellent nurses did not pass the NCLEX the first time around for one reason or another, so don't be afraid to try again.

One exceptional nurse I know failed not once, but *twice*! Most would have concluded nursing was not in the cards and thrown in the towel, but she didn't give up. She learned as much as she could about the testing process, maintained her focus and most importantly, kept a positive attitude. She did not let the test results define her - rather, she used them as a tool to improve her performance.

Use the Diagnostic Profile to help you prepare, keep your chin up and maintain your focus. Ask one of your instructors about tutoring, or enroll in a review course. Devote a realistic amount of time each day to preparation and studies. You got through nursing school - you can pass this test!

And my friend who failed the NCLEX twice? She finally passed on her third attempt. A self-professed NCLEX professional, she now devotes her time to helping others pass the exam, in addition to maintaining a successful career as a registered nurse. One of her patients was so impressed with her that he developed a nursing scholarship fund in her honor. How's that for an inspirational finish? If she can do it, so can you!

Graduate School

You may decide at some point in your career that you would like to expand the scope of your practice and responsibilities. Graduate school allows you to pursue an advanced degree focusing specialization in the clinical area of your choosing. Advanced practice nurses enjoy significantly higher earnings, increased professional autonomy and greater personal satisfaction with their careers.

Areas of advanced practice you can pursue via master's degree or advanced practice nursing certification programs include:

Clinical Nurse Specialist

A clinical nurse specialist has advanced training concentrating on a specific area of nursing. They function as expert clinicians, educators, consultants and researchers, exhibiting mastery of the principles of treatment and care in the clinical area of their choosing. You can be a clinical nurse specialist in almost any area of nursing, although the practice is generally hospital-based. Examples include critical care, oncology, geriatric, education, staff development, acute adult care, emergency, medical-surgical, immunology, etc.

Community Health Nursing

Community health nurses focus on improving the health of communities as a whole, and subgroups within a community population. They assess the health needs of population groups, develop and evaluate community-based programs, design nursing interventions and coordinate the delivery of community health nursing services.

Nurse Anesthetist

Nurse anesthesia practice is based on a continuum of care to provide anesthesia services before, during and after surgical and obstetrical procedures, including patient assessment and monitoring.

Nurse Educator

Nurse educators are teachers. Their training prepares them to devise, implement and evaluate clinical practicum, classroom instructional strategies and curriculum design. They work as staff development specialists and nursing instructors.

Nurse Midwife

Nurse midwives provide primary health care for women and newborns with an emphasis on normal pregnancy, labor and delivery. They also provide services for well gynecology and family planning care.

Nurse Practitioner

Nurse practitioners are educated to assess, counsel, diagnose, prescribe and manage the care of their patients, in collaboration with other healthcare professionals. They focus on management of health and illness, teaching and counseling, and coordinating care. Nurse practitioners specialize in the area of their choosing. Examples include pediatrics, acute adult care, gerontology, primary care and family practice, community health, emergency, critical care, etc.

Nursing Informatics

The nursing informatics specialty focuses on the structure and process of nursing information as it supports the practice of nursing. It is a combination of computer science, information science and nursing science that includes the development, analysis and evaluation of the systems and technology that are used to manage patient care.

Nursing Management

Nursing management prepares you to assume executive positions in a wide range of health care organizations, consulting firms and corporations. Integrating the disciplines of nursing and business management, this specialty area focuses on health care systems, business issues and management accountability as applied to nursing care delivery. Dual MSN/MBA degree programs are available.

Research Nursing

Research nurses conduct and coordinate clinical research to positively impact patient outcomes and service delivery. They are involved in the research process areas as project managers, consultants, educators or adverse event coordinators.

Why Become a Nurse Practitioner?

The biggest factor in my decision to become a nurse practitioner was to expand my horizons and further my nursing career. I was no longer satisfied with staff nursing and wanted to advance to a leadership role. Management is not something I am interested in, but being a nurse is. So naturally, specializing in critical care as a nurse practitioner will satisfy my need to function as a nurse in a leadership role.

- Sally Villasenor, BA, BSN, TNCC
1996 graduate of Wayne State University

As you can see, there are many options for advanced practice if you decide to take your career to the next level. Also, graduate schools tend to be more flexible when it comes to accommodating working professionals. RN to MSN accelerated bridge programs are very popular, and distance learning opportunities are abundant.

For more information on graduate schools and advanced practice, visit out website.

Transitioning to Work

You survived nursing school, passed the NCLEX and now you have your license in hand. Hard to believe, isn't it? The reality that you are a licensed nurse takes a while to sink in. YOU are a NURSE!

You've worked hard to get where you are - that piece of paper represents years of dedication, blood, sweat and tears. Now it's time to leave the security of nursing school and go out into the real world. It's time to find your first nursing job.

You went to school with a specific goal in mind, so you don't want just any job - you want to find your *dream* job. Every job has its pluses and minuses; there is no such thing as the perfect job. Realistically, your dream job is one that offers a good fit for your skills, career goals and personal interests. You are looking for a position and work environment that will lend itself to a fulfilling professional career, while also allowing opportunities for personal growth and development.

Take some time to really think about what you are looking for:
- ✦ Is there a specialty area you want to practice in? Will you need to gain general experience first? What facilities in your area offer opportunities for both?
- ✦ What are your scheduling desires? Do you have children or a significant other? Do you have a preference about days or nights? Fulltime, part time or fill-in work?
- ✦ What environment is best suited to you? The hospital setting? Community clinics? Long term care facilities? Family practice offices?
- ✦ Is there are certain facility you already want to work for? If so, do they have opportunities inline with your career goals? Are there steps you can take to increase your chances of getting hired there (volunteer work, industry contacts, additional experience or certification)?
- ✦ What are the requirements of the type of job you are looking for? Do you meet these requirements, and if not, what can you do to change that?
- ✦ Where do you want to be 5 years from now? Map out a plan to get there and follow it.

Put thought into your decisions. Make sure you are making choices that support your goals and needs.

The most important advice I can give you is this:
> *Do not automatically accept the first job you are offered.*

Don't be afraid to shop around. You're anxious to get started, and the need for income is a high priority, but so is your commitment to your career and your future employer. Job-hopping is deadly for new grads, so make sure your first job is one you will be happy with for a while.

Finding Your Dream Job

Great ideas need landing gear as well as wings.

- C. D. Jackson

The first key to finding your dream job is knowing where to look. Many people assume the classified ads in their local newspaper are the best place to find jobs. Not necessarily! Many of the "best" jobs are never advertised.

Where, then, can you find these top-notch jobs that are a new nurse's dream? Here are some great sources you can use to get your search underway:

✦ **Friends and Industry Contacts**
  Tap the people you know - ask around about job openings and find out which facilities have a good reputation in your area. Networking is free and an inside referral can give you an advantage when interviewing with top employers.

✦ **College Placement Office**
  Your college placement office is there to help you find a job. Industry recruiters collaborate with colleges to fill openings, and your placement office will have a comprehensive listing of local jobs specifically suited to new grads. Additionally, they will offer career counseling and can help you with resume writing and interview techniques.

✦ **Professional Associations**
  Any of the student or professional organizations you belong to will have career resources you can take advantage of, including job listings. Get in touch with the local contact person to inquire about job openings in your area.

✦ **Recruiting and Placement Firms**
  There are many recruiting and placement firms specializing in the healthcare industry. You can find them in your local phone book under "Employment Agencies." These companies will contact employers for you and help you get an interview. You should not be charged a fee for this service. Recruiting agencies typically earn a commission from the employer, *not* the candidate, when a match is made which results in employment.

Other great resources you can check with include your state employment services office, the federal government and the internet. So you see, the classified ads are not the only place to find jobs. Investigate your options and widen your search so you don't miss out on a really great job!

Resumes

A well-written cover letter and a top-quality resume are essential to getting an interview. Employers almost always have more applicants than they have time to meet with, so only those individuals whose resumes stand out will be called in for an interview. You need to make a good impression - it's critical.

First, let's cover the basics.

DO:

- ✦ Make it look professional - use nice paper and good print quality.
- ✦ Keep it simple - clean margins, basic fonts (Times New Roman, Arial, Helvetica), black ink.
- ✦ Pay attention to grammar, spelling and punctuation. Your resume and cover letter should be error-free, so proofread it several times.
- ✦ Have your contact information on every page, in case they get separated.

DON'T:

- ✦ Use fancy fonts, colored ink, graphics or colored paper (other than neutral colors, such as off-white, beige and grey).
- ✦ Rely only on your computer's spellchecker - have friends proof your work.
- ✦ Use poor-quality photocopies - it looks bad.
- ✦ Use generic cover letters.

Each resume you send out should include a personalized cover letter specific to that employer and job. Things you should include in the cover letter are:

- ✦ What job you are applying for and how you heard about it.
- ✦ Why you are interested in the job.
- ✦ Why you feel you are good fit for the position.
- ✦ A brief summary of your experience or training.
- ✦ Your salary requirements.
- ✦ How you can be contacted.
- ✦ A *thank you*.

When writing your resume, keep it brief - 2 pages maximum. Things you should include:

- ◆ Name, contact information and *nursing licensure number*.
- ◆ Career Objective - one to two lines defining what you are looking for.
- ◆ Experience - start with your most recent job first, and briefly summarize your job duties and responsibilities.
- ◆ Education - list the high school and college(s) you have attended; include dates and degrees earned, special honors, etc.
- ◆ Additional Training and Certification.
- ◆ Honors and Awards.
- ◆ Professional Affiliations.
- ◆ Volunteer activities.

SAMPLE COVER LETTER

Jane Nurse, RN
123 Maple Street
Your Town, CA 90210
(123) 456-7890

June 10, 2001

Mr. Joe Recruiter
Director of Human Resources
Big Time Hospital
456 Broadway
Los Angeles, CA 90200

Dear Mr. Recruiter,

I am writing in response to your advertisement in the June 10, 2001 edition of the Los Angeles Times for a Medical-Surgical RN. Big Time Hospital has an outstanding reputation as a community-centered healthcare facility, and I am very interested in joining your team.

I am a recent graduate of Best Nursing School of America and am looking for a position in the medical-surgical area. I am seeking a salary in the range of $28,000 - $32,000 per year. I received high quality training and significant clinical experience through the nursing program, graduating with honors. Additionally, I have 3 years' experience as a medical technician in the healthcare field.

I believe I would be a good fit for this position and a valuable asset to your team. My background in the healthcare field and clinical training meet your qualifications for this position. Additionally, I am an excellent communicator, detail-oriented and possess solid time management skills.

I would appreciate the opportunity to discuss in person how I can contribute to the success of Big Time Hospital. I have enclosed my resume for your review and am available for an interview at your convenience. I can be reached at (123) 456-7890. I look forward to speaking with you.

Best regards,

Jane Nurse, RN

Tip

Your resume should not include a section pertaining to personal information (such as married, 2 kids, etc.). This type of data is not related to your suitability for the job. Keep the focus on what skills and experience you have that make you the right match for the position.

By paying attention to details and keeping your focus on what qualifies you for the job, you can write a cover letter and resume that stand out in the crowd. Making a good first impression goes a long way towards getting called in for an interview.

Interviewing

Your resume worked - you've just been scheduled for an interview. Fantastic! Now what do you do? You *research*. Do your homework on the potential employer. Find out about the company, the facility, and the programs they offer - learn as much as you can. Why? So you will be better able to ask questions during the interview process, of course.

"What?" you say, "That's not the way it works...the employer asks YOU the questions - not the other way around."

Not so. Who ever said the interview process is a one-way street? While your potential employer is evaluating you, you should also be evaluating *them*. Remember, it's not about getting *"a"* job - it's about getting *"the"* job - one that meets your criteria and goals. Here are some things you may want to ask about during the interview:

+ Orientation - How many weeks does the orientation last? How do they approach training new employees? Attempt to assess if they have a solid training program in place.
+ Scheduling - Is there mandatory overtime? Required float assignments? Is the schedule set or does it change from week to week?
+ Staffing - What are the minimum nurse to patient ratios for your unit? How do they utilize unlicensed personnel (such as CNAs)? How do they handle shortages (agency nurses, voluntary overtime)?
+ Certification - Do they offer on-site training and certification for specialty units?
+ Evaluation - How are new employees evaluated and how often?
+ Development - What opportunities are available for professional development, continuing education and advancement? Do they provide the kind of training and advancement opportunities you need to meet your career goals?

These questions will give you more to go on so you can make an informed choice if the position is offered to you. Additionally, asking questions during the interview shows that you are interested and proactive.

"Wait a second...didn't you forget one? What about pay and benefits?"

Good question. It's generally considered a faux-pas for the applicant to bring up the subject of pay during an interview - let the interviewer bring it up (and they *will* bring it up). As far as benefits go, these will be addressed when an offer of employment is made. You can ask any questions related to benefits at that time.

When you are interviewing, you will most likely meet with several people. This can occur during one meeting or over the course of several meetings - probably at least *two* interviews. The first will be with the human resources professional. If that meeting is successful, you may be called back to meet with the director of nursing and the charge nurse for your intended area. Don't let this intimidate you - stay positive, keep calm and just be yourself.

They will ask you fairly typical questions you can prepare for in advance, such as why you are interested in this job, why you would be the best choice and what your career goals are. Think about these questions before you start interviewing so you can plan for how you will answer them.

Don't Panic

You also may be asked questions you are not prepared for, or questions that are always difficult to answer. Things like, "What are your weaknesses?" or questions that deal with case scenarios - "What would you do in this situation?" The key here is to take a moment to center yourself - it is perfectly okay to take a moment to collect your thoughts so you can answer in the best possible way.

What Do Recruiters Look For In A Candidate?

Independent recruiters and human resource professionals both agree on what to look for in a potential candidate.

✦ Whether you are a new grad or an experienced nurse, always keep in mind that old adage, "First appearances are important." Invest in a coordinated, neutral tone, business-like outfit that flatters your body type.

✦ Prepare a list of questions about the facility and job. Take this list with you in a notebook and keep it handy for reference, as well as for taking notes along the way.

✦ Equally important is to prepare a list of questions you will most likely be asked and practice your answers. What interests you most about the opportunity? What do you feel qualifies you for this position? What are your personal and professional goals for the next year (and beyond)? What are your proudest achievements - personally and professionally? What are your strengths? Weaknesses?

✦ Do not ask about benefits until you're offered the job.

✦ Never state a specific salary requirement. Keep this "open for discussion" verbally, as well as on any personnel form.

Beyond the basic requirements of the position, the interviewer is always looking for candidates that exhibit good interpersonal skills - good eye contact, good verbal skills, good preparation and not easily flustered by a negative question.

There have never been more opportunities for nurses at all levels. However, getting the specific job you want takes solid preparation. Both professional recruiters and human resource representatives will only recommend onward in the interview process those candidates that project an image of professionalism and readiness for the job.

- Pat Erickson, President and Owner
Erickson & Associates, Inc. Advanced Practice Nurse Search Consultants

*Salaries, Benefits & Perks**

What is the standard starting salary for new grads? What benefits are the norm? Knowing what is typical for your area can help you when you begin to evaluate job offers.

For new RNs, the national average starting salary is about $15.41 an hour. For LPNs, it is $11.65 an hour. These figures will be higher or lower depending on such factors as location and the type of facility you are applying to. Regionally, entry level nursing wages are as follows:*

Registered Nurses

New England	$17.30	South Central	$13.98
Middle Atlantic	$16.12	Mountain	$14.71
South Atlantic	$14.62	Pacific	$17.69
North Central	$15.52		

Licensed Practical Nurses

New England	$14.12	South Central	$10.45
Middle Atlantic	$12.39	Mountain	$10.77
South Atlantic	$11.05	Pacific	$13.28
North Central	$10.69		

*Nursing 2000 Salary Survey, Springhouse Publishing

As far as practice area, hospitals pay the best, followed very closely by home health care. Rehabilitation centers and sub-acute care pay the least, followed by longterm care facilities. Earnings increase overall with advanced training, certification and experience.

The initial hourly wage is called your base rate. Depending on your employer, you may be offered differential pay - an extra amount added onto your base rate. The most common type of differential pay is known as shift differential, which is paid for working nights. Hospitals in particular may add an extra $1.00 an hour or more to your pay if you work the night shift. Other types of differential pay include holiday and call-in differentials (if you are called in to work on your day off), and less commonly, certification differential - extra pay based on specialized training or certification

Your salary is not the "be-all-end-all" it would appear to be. Sometimes, a lower than average salary is offset by a fantastic benefits program. The most common benefits offered are insurances: health, vision, dental, life, disability, liability, etc. Also common are tuition reimbursement programs, onsite certification/training and retirement plans.

Employers may also offer less common benefits, often referred to as "perks," to attract and keep qualified employees. These can include: free parking, meal discounts, on-site childcare, fitness facilities, employee assistance programs, credit unions, and flexible scheduling.

Flexible scheduling options are becoming very popular. You may find some places offering 4 days on, followed by 3 days off, giving you a full week's pay plus a three-day weekend. To encourage weekend staffing, some employers will offer a full week's pay for working *just* the weekend, or the weekend plus one day. Not too shabby! Still other facilities may allow you to create your own schedule - what could be better than that?

It is important here to look at the whole package - you need to consider the combination of pay, benefits and perks to truly evaluate what is being offered. Sometimes, differential pay or a simple benefit that will make your life easier will be the determining factor between two equal job offers.

Evaluating Job Offers

One you have aced a couple of interviews, you will begin to receive job offers. Remember, you don't have to take the first job offered to you and most organizations do not expect you to make an immediate decision. Consider all your options and make the best choice for you. When evaluating job offers, you need to look at:

◆ **The Organization**
What is its reputation? Does it have a solid background or has it been plagued with financial difficulties and/or high employee turnover? Does the organization's mission match your values and ideals?

◆ **The Facility**
Is the location good for you? How long is the commute? Are the building, grounds and equipment well-maintained (if not, it could indicate financial problems)? Is size a factor (i.e. do you prefer a small practice setting or a large hospital)? What is the atmosphere? How is employee morale?

◆ **The Job**
Is the job what you are looking for? Are the job duties in-line with your background, experience and goals? Would you enjoy the work? Are the staffing ratios safe? What about the hours and schedule? Are flexible scheduling options available?

✦ Pay and Benefits

Is the pay comparable to other facilities in the area? What benefits are offered and what is the employee portion of the cost? What perks are offered?

✦ Opportunities

Does the facility encourage professional development? Are there advancement opportunities? Onsite training and certification in specialty areas? What about tuition reimbursement?

✦ Career Ladder

Is there an established plan to progressively recognize your training/experience? **Career ladder** is such a program. In it, nurses are promoted along "steps" (Clinical Nurse I, Clinical Nurse II etc.) as their education and/or experience advances.

The most important thing to consider is your gut feeling. How does it feel to you? An organization may meet all your requirements, but if you still feel something is off or you are not quite comfortable, it's best to pass on it.

When evaluating employers, keep in mind your longterm goals and make sure you will be able to go in the direction you want. You will have this first job for several years, so do everything you can ahead of time to make sure it is the best job for you.

The First Six Months

As you prepare to embark on your new nursing career, you will probably feel a combination of emotions: fear, excitement, anxiety, joy. You know you have done everything in your power to prepare for this day, but if you are honest with yourself, you probably don't feel *nearly* ready enough.

Nothing can truly prepare you for the nursing experience, but knowing some things ahead of time will make the transition easier. This section is devoted to things you don't learn in nursing school. My hope is to prepare you for the reality shock so you can move forward with greater peace of mind. Included are tips and suggestions for making your transition as smooth as possible, and helpful advice you can use to become the best nurse you can be.

Learning Does Not End With School

The most vital thing for new nurses to know is this: Learning does not end with school. School knowledge (book smarts) is merely the framework for your nursing career to build itself around. Your personal experiences with each new patient, doctor, seasoned and novice nurse alike, will be your school once you graduate. A motivated nurse thrives on this continual learning that I like to call "being a perpetual student." No, you won't be assigned any "homework" or "nursing process papers," but don't be surprised if you find yourself subscribing to and reading nursing journals, looking up pathophysiology and drugs you are not familiar with, going above and beyond the call of duty just to be informed. Be proud of your decision to be a nurse - the possibilities and specialties are endless!

- Sally Villasenor, BA, BSN, TNNC
1996 graduate of Wayne State University

You Really ARE Ready!

We don't know who we are until we see what we can do.

- Martha Grimes

Believe it or not, *every* new graduate is nervous - even those who outwardly appear confident and ready to take on the world. It is absolutely normal for you to feel that you are not ready. Just remember that you are! You have already learned and demonstrated all the basic competencies expected of an entry-level nurse. As nursing instructors say, *"All the knowledge you need is in your head - now transfer it to your hands."*

The first six months of nursing will be nerve-wracking. You will be learning the ropes at your new facility, as well as settling in to your role as a licensed professional. Without the safety net of your clinical instructor, procedures you were once confident about may now seem problematic. The issue is not your abilities - it's your comfort level with the responsibility connected to your actions. There is no one there to give you the "okay" when you make a decision. Suddenly, routine tasks take on new significance, as you realize you are ultimately responsible for your patient's well-being.

The only way to overcome these self-doubts is to give yourself time. Most new nurses don't feel comfortable with their role until they have been practicing for a year or more. You need time to adjust and acclimate to your surroundings, to become familiar with standard protocols and procedures. You need time to find your voice and confidence as a professional.

Take comfort in knowing that you are not alone in your fears, and that you really do have the skills and knowledge to do this. Your concerns are normal. Don't be too hard on yourself, and be prepared to learn from your mistakes. Confidence will come with time and experience.

The Preceptor Relationship

> *The trouble with most of us is that we would rather*
> *be ruined by praise than saved by criticism.*
>
> *- Norman Vincent Peale*

At your new job, you will participate in an orientation program that can last anywhere from three weeks to three months. During this time, you will be guided by one or more preceptors who will serve as mentors and advisors as you transition to the professional role.

It is important to develop a good working relationship with your preceptor. Be open to suggestions and constructive criticism, and use your active listening skills. You can learn a lot from your preceptor, if you are receptive to their guidance.

Some things to keep in mind:

✦ **Don't take criticism personally**

It is not *you* they are critiquing - it is your actions or technique. They are trying to help you, not discourage you. Listen with an open mind and use their suggestions to become a better nurse.

✦ **Be honest**

Don't try to cover up mistakes or say you know how to do something when you don't. No one expects you to know everything right away. For nurses, learning is a lifelong process.

✦ **Step up to the plate**

Don't be afraid to take on responsibility. Be willing to give new things a try, and work on becoming a contributing member of the team.

✦ **Ask questions!**
Your preceptor is there to answer questions and expects you to ask for clarification or help when you need it. They will be more concerned if you don't have any questions. It's natural to have many, many questions in the first six months.

✦ **Be gracious**
Most of the time, your preceptor has his or her own patient case load and responsibilities to attend to, in addition to mentoring and helping you. Respect their time and be appreciative of their assistance.

Work with your preceptor to become the best nurse you can. Stay positive and put effort into developing a good working relationship. Your preceptor is an invaluable resource who will foster enormous personal and professional growth. Take full advantage of the time you have with them and let yourself soar!

Legal Mumbo Jumbo

One thing many new nurses are not prepared for is the legal reality of being a licensed professional. Yes, you learned about it in class, but suddenly having all that responsibility squarely on your shoulders can be unsettling, to say the least. The potential for lawsuits is very real, so you need to be informed about your rights and responsibilities.

There are two kinds of laws pertaining to nursing practice:
Nurse Practice Acts (NPAs) are laws in each state that are instrumental in defining the scope of nursing practice. NPAs protect public health, safety, and welfare. This protection includes shielding the public from unqualified and unsafe nurses, and as such, NPAs are arguably the most important pieces of legislation related to nursing practice.

In each state, statutory law directs entry into nursing practice, defines the scope of practice, and establishes disciplinary procedures. State boards of nursing oversee this statutory law. They have the responsibility and authority to protect the public by determining who is competent to practice nursing.

Common Law is derived from principles or social mores rather than from rules and regulations. It consists of broad, interpretive principles based on reason, traditional justice and common sense.

Together, the NPAs and Common Law define nursing practice.

Tip

It is a nurse's responsibility to be informed on both the NPA and Common Law for the state(s) in which they are licensed to practice. It is critical for students and nurses need to be aware of the legal issues pertaining to the profession. Familiarity with the law and relevant court rulings helps in understanding the scope of practice and responsibilities that come with being a licensed caregiver, as well as providing insight on how to prevent legal problems before they happen.

A few more bits of advice:

✦ **Never accept an unsafe assignment**
You have a legal and ethical obligation not to accept an unsafe patient load (more patients than you are able to adequately care for) or an assignment requiring care you are not qualified or competent to give (anything outside your scope of practice and training). It's your license on the line here - if you accept such an assignment and something goes wrong, you will be subject to discipline for incompetence or negligence. You could lose your license and you may be held personally responsible for damages. The judicial system will not care that you were "just helping out" during a staffing shortage, and neither will the board of nursing. Most importantly, remember that you have an ethical responsibility to protect your patients - that is your top priority.

✦ **Document everything**
Keep accurate, objective records when charting, and watch the details - it may save you later on.

✦ **Keep your eyes open and communicate any concerns**
The two most common reasons for lawsuits are failure to monitor and failure to advise. Make time to check on your patients and always call the physician if you have any concerns. Keep the communication flowing with your patients and with their physicians - it is critical.

Read up on the NPA for your state so you will know your responsibilities and limitations. Subscribe to professional nursing journals to stay abreast of the latest court rulings. Protect yourself - this is one reality you cannot afford to ignore.

Point of View: Legal Issues in Nursing
What are the legal aspects of patient confidentiality?
Essentially, all healthcare providers not directly involved in the care of the patient must have the patient's permission to access their information. The only exception is third party contracts or as otherwise allowed by law, particularly at the state level. Failure to respect the patient's right to confidentiality and privacy may expose the nurse to individual liability. For example, the nurse could be liable if found disclosing medical conditions of patients to friends, colleagues, media, etc., or disclosing sensitive lab results to non-health care providers. Sometimes confidential information may be disclosed, particularly if such information could cause serious harm to the patient, the family or staff. An example would be in cases of suspected child, spouse or elder abuse, or threats of suicide by a patient.

How important is it to carry liability insurance?

I strongly recommend carrying liability insurance as a nurse. If I were involved or named in any action, I would want to ensure my best professional interests were considered and protected to the extent possible. Increasingly, more nurses are being named individually in suits, and may work in undesirable conditions that may predispose them to being named. Additionally, the nursing scope of practice has become more autonomous and more technical than in the past. Despite having some liability coverage from the hospital or facility, I still would want to be represented on my own behalf. It is a small price to pay for what could be devastating consequences.

Can nurses get sued?

In the cases I have reviewed, the most common reasons nurses are named in suits involve medication errors, failure to perform a nursing procedure correctly, failure to notify or communicate changes in a patient's status, failure to prevent falls and patient injuries, failure to invoke the chain of command, and inappropriate use or misuse of restraints. The individual nurse can do several things to prevent these events from occurring, and many involve common sense, such as:

✦ Know your strengths and weaknesses or limitations in knowledge or experience.

✦ Know and follow the hospital policies and procedures .

✦ Adhere to the "five rights" of medication administration.

✦ Provide timely and accurate documentation of care.

✦ Keep the chain of command in mind and delegate the appropriate patient care activities.

✦ Remain current and competent in the area of practice (by continuing education, skills validation, competency assessments, certification, reading journals, etc.).

You will reduce your exposure to liability if you always apply the nursing process principles, maintain good rapport with patients and, when short on time, focus on what really makes a difference in patient outcome.

- Vickie L. Milazzo, RN, MSN, JD
President, Medical-Legal Consulting Institute, Inc.

Tip

One more thing to think about - liability insurance. Most employers will offer employer-sponsored liability and malpractice insurance to cover you, but you may want to consider taking out an extra policy of your own. The American Nurses Association offers supplemental coverage that is very affordable if you do not have an insurance provider of your own.

bandidobooks.com

Contact your state board of nursing for more information (see Resources for contact information), or visit our web site. There you will find links to the state boards of nursing, for easy access the information you need.

I Wish They Would Have Told Me...

Your first six months in the field will be an enormous learning curve. No doubt about it, there are just some things they don't teach you in nursing school. In situations like these, a little inside information is just what the nurse ordered...so here is the real scoop on things you need to know.

MEDICAL-SURGICAL OR SPECIALTY UNIT?

There are advantages and disadvantages to the unit where you first choose to work. Traditional wisdom holds that new grads need one year of medical-surgical experience before going on to a specialty unit.

Medical Surgical Unit	
Benefits	**Drawbacks**
✦ Best way for overall experience	✦ Higher nurse-patient ratios
✦ Exposure to a variety of cases	✦ No specialization
✦ Lower stress level for new grads	✦ It may not be your "dream" job

Medical-surgical experience is sometimes required before you can transfer to a specialty unit, and it's the best way to build your confidence in basic care, since you are exposed to such a wide variety of conditions.

So what of going straight to a specialty unit right out of school?

Specialty Unit	
Benefits	**Drawbacks**
✦ Matches your interests	✦ High stress level of new grads
✦ Challenging work	✦ May not be a good fit
✦ Certification in specialty area	✦ Lack of general experience
✦ Fast track to career goals.	✦ May not be open to new grads

Unlike in previous eras where medical-surgical experience was the rule, new nurses now have a much easier time obtaining residency in the area of nursing they are want. If you are flexible about shift, location and pay, you will have much better chances of getting into a specialty unit right out of school.

Watch Out

A word of caution, however - it is hard enough learning the basic ropes of nursing, without having to learn specialization at the same time. This can be very stressful for new grads, and can affect your confidence. Moreover, many specialty units now require a contractual agreement to work there for a minimum period of time. If you get into that situation and find you don't like the work, you will be stuck. What it all boils down to is a personal choice. Think about the pro's and con's of each option, then decide what will work best for you.

WORK THE NIGHT SHIFT OR NOT?

A willingness to work the night shift will open a lot of doors for finding a position in the facility and area your prefer, and the pay is better. On the flip side, it can wreck havoc on your physiology and social life.

Night Shift	
Benefits	**Drawbacks**
✦ Differential pay	✦ Loss of natural biorhythm
✦ Better choice of units	✦ Hard on outside relationships
✦ Less bureaucracy, more autonomy	✦ Career stall (harder to get noticed by administration)

If you choose to work nights, here is some advice to help make it easier:

- ✦ Schedule your night shifts back to back, and try to switch to your family's natural cycle during clusters of days off.
- ✦ Use room-darkening shades, black-out curtains, and a white noise machine to help make daytime sleep more like night time.
- ✦ Don't go to sleep immediately after your shift - allow time to unwind, just as if you had a day job.
- ✦ Schedule daytime appointments and errands in the morning, as close to the end of your shift as possible.
- ✦ Use a digital watch with military time to help with charting.
- ✦ Bring healthy snacks to work - avoid the vending machines. You don't want to have a low-blood sugar moment at 4:00 a.m.
- ✦ Take a 5-minute break to step outside or walk the halls if you feel yourself getting drowsy.
- ✦ Make time for good nutrition, adequate sleep, exercise and family - your career is important, but it is not your life.

Working nights does not have to be awful - in fact, many nurses prefer it. Night shift crews tend to be closer-knit and often work together better than their dayshift counterparts.

The key is to determine if it will work for you. Evaluate your options and make a choice you can live with - that's the bottom line.

UNION OR NON-UNION?

Unions are becoming more popular in the nursing profession. As a new nurse, you may not have had exposure to unions, so a little primer is in order.

Unions serve to represent a group of nurses by presenting a unified front to management on group issues. They negotiate raises and benefits, mediate problems, and monitor such things as safe staffing and working conditions.

Union membership requires the payment of annual dues and participation in actions voted upon by members (i.e., strikes). The intent is to promote better working conditions for nurses by presenting a united voice to management, but some nurses may find they are not comfortable with the politics of it. Union effectiveness varies - it all boils down to the participation of its members and, more importantly, the leadership representing the group. Are the leaders active? Do members support the leaders they have chosen? These are important factors to investigate.

Unions	
Benefits	**Drawbacks**
◆ Solidarity	◆ No voice as an individual
◆ Better wages and benefits	◆ Jobs awarded by seniority
◆ Better staffing ratios	◆ Hard to get rid of bad nurses
◆ Mediation	◆ Strikes
◆ Works best with large organizations (300+)	◆ Not as effective with small organizations (less than 300)

When you have to decide between joining a union or staying solo, learn as much as you can about the history and direction of the union in question. How do they operate? How successful have they been? How content are the members? Also, think about your own personal beliefs and values. Are you comfortable letting someone speak for you? Are you willing to stick with it during a walk-out? Do you agree with this method of interaction with administration?

As with everything else in nursing, it comes down to a personal choice - what is best for you?

VIOLENCE IN THE WORKPLACE

Violence in the workplace is concern faced by all healthcare professionals. When you are dealing with a diverse population of patients who may be frightened, emotionally volatile, mentally ill or under the influence of alcohol and drugs, the potential for physical assault is very real. Most frequently seen in the hospital and mental health settings, nurses routinely deal with violence perpetrated by unstable patients. Kicking, hitting, slapping, pinching, spitting and verbal abuse occur much more often than you would think.

Being aware of this potentiality is your best defense:

+ Keep alert, use your head and avoid volatile situations.
+ Diffuse escalating situations - try to see what your patients see, feel what they feel - try to understand so you can adjust your actions to be less threatening or frightening.
+ Never wear your stethoscope around your neck when bending over patients, and never turn your back on someone who has been verbally abusive or who appears unstable.
+ If you are at all uncomfortable with a situation, get assistance right away - better to be safe than sorry.

Listen to your instincts - they won't steer you wrong. When it comes to workplace violence, you need to be proactive so you can protect yourself *and* your patients from harm.

MORE THINGS YOU NEED TO KNOW

There are other things you need to be prepared for when you enter the nursing workforce, certain realities that come with the territory, but about which you may not be aware.

What are some of the "surprises" new nurses face? Here's a list of things you may encounter - better to know now than be thrown for a loop later.

Top 10 "Surprises" New Nurses May Experience

1. Mandatory overtime

Some facilities routinely <u>require</u> overtime.

2. Required floating

Many hospitals require float days, where you are sent to unfamiliar units to cover staffing shortages.

3. High nurse to patient ratios

Normal medical-surgical ratios are 1:6 days, 1:8 nights; some places are as high as 1:10 days, 1:14 nights!

4. No lunch breaks

Eat when you can - you won't get a full 30 minutes most days due to the nature of the work.

5. Working on your days off

Call-ins are common when understaffing occurs. This can be avoided by unplugging your phone.

6. Nurses eating their young

This is not always the case of course, but nurses have a notorious reputation for not supporting their newest members.

7. Toxic work environments

I am not referring to chemicals, here - by this, I mean negative energy. Every place has it share of burnt-out employees, disgruntled workers and gossipmongers. Don't get drawn into it - stay positive and avoid the negative people.

8. Hostile Physicians

I do not wish to stereotype here, as there are many fantastic physicians who are compassionate, excellent clinicians and maintain good relationships with other members of the healthcare team. However, you need to be aware that *some* physicians are difficult to work with.

9. Pharmacology Exam for New Employees

Some facilities require new nurses to pass a pharmacology exam before they are allowed to pass medications. You can do this, obviously - but it might come as a surprise, which is why I have brought it up.

10. Taking your Work Home with You

The last item on this list is inevitable for new nurses - it is extremely difficult to leave work at work when you are talking about real people whose lives are on the line. You may find yourself unable to stop thinking about a patient who died on your watch, or a child who is not expected to make it through the night. You may find yourself retracing your steps in your mind, trying to figure out what more you could have done. Part of being a caregiver is caring, so it comes with the territory, but you will have to develop a way to keep your job from taking over your life.

Teamwork

You will always be shorthanded. Don't complain about what you can't get done; instead, work on ways to get it all done with the team. The most helpful thing is for nurses to work together for the common good of all patients, not just their own.

- Sandy Martin, LPN
RN student, Lehigh Carbon Community College

NURSING SUPERSTITIONS

Every profession has its own set of superstitions or unwritten rules. Nursing is no exception. There is a standing code that has been passed down from one generation of nurses to the next, and it is time now to pass the torch along to you.

Top 3 Unwritten Rules of Nursing

1. Never, EVER utter the "Q" word.
Don't say, "Boy, it sure is quiet tonight!" That is the ultimate kiss of death in nursing. Doing so guarantees that disaster will strike, most likely within 10 minutes.

2. Never utter the name of your most dreaded patient aloud.
Casually bringing up the name of your most difficult patient is akin to calling him on the phone and asking him to visit. He will, without a doubt, show up within 30 minutes.

3. Watch out for the full moon.
Nursing lore has it that full moons and periods of low barometric pressure bring out the crazies, spawn natural catastrophes and guarantee a full house.

Keep these three rules in mind, and you'll fit right in!

FINAL WORDS OF ADVICE
You are standing on the threshold of a learning adventure and the career of a lifetime. Nursing, despite its challenges, is rewarding and deeply satisfying work. It's about making a difference, every single day.

Final advice for you to help you on your way:

◆ Don't let anyone intimidate you or make you feel somehow less than you are.

◆ Work at work, but take care of yourself and your family at home. Don't let work overshadow the other parts of your life.

◆ Allow yourself to feel. It's okay to cry with your patients - it does not make you any less professional. You are human, too.

◆ Know that the majority of mistakes new nurses make are not life-threatening. Be honest, learn from your mistakes and move on - don't dwell on things.

◆ Don't undermine your confidence with negative self-talk. It will take at least a year to reach your comfort zone - allow yourself time to learn.

◆ Find mentors in addition to your preceptor - nurses you can call on when you are in a bind or need help.

◆ Ask questions - lots of questions!

◆ Listen to your instincts - the longer you are a nurse, the more developed they will become - and they will rarely be wrong.

And finally,

Always remember that your patients are human beings first and foremost. Treat them with dignity, consideration, compassion and respect.

Keep your empathy, keep your focus, and keep your sense of humor. Be the best nurse you can be!

Resources

The following pages list resources and organizations that may be helpful to you on your path to nursing. All contact information is current as of the date of publication. For more resources, check out our web site!

State Boards of Nursing

National Council of State Boards of Nursing
676 N. St. Clair Street, Suite 550
Chicago, Illinois, 60611-2921
(312) 787-6555

Alabama Board of Nursing
770 Washington Avenue
RSA Plaza, Ste 250
Montgomery, AL 36130-3900
Phone: (334) 242-4060

Alabama Board of Nursing
770 Washington Avenue
RSA Plaza, Ste 250
Montgomery, AL 36130-3900
Phone: (334) 242-4060

Alaska Board of Nursing
Dept. of Comm. & Econ. Development
Div. of Occupational Licensing
3601 C Street, Suite 722
Anchorage, AK 99503
Phone: (907) 269-8161

American Samoa Health Services
Services Regulatory Board
LBJ Tropical Medical Center
Pago Pago, AS 96799
Phone: (684) 633-1222

Connecticut Board of Examiners for Nursing
Dept. of Public Health
410 Capitol Avenue, MS# 13PHO
P.O. Box 340308
Hartford, CT 06134-0328
Phone: (860) 509-7624

Arizona State Board of Nursing
1651 E. Morten Avenue, Suite 210
Phoenix, AZ 85020
Phone: (602) 331-8111

Arkansas State Board of Nursing
University Tower Building
1123 S. University, Suite 800
Little Rock, AR 72204-1619
Phone: (501) 686-2700

California Board of Registered Nursing
400 R St., Ste. 4030
Sacramento, CA 95814-6239
Phone: (916) 322-3350

California Board of Vocational Nurse and Psychiatric Technician Examiners
2535 Capitol Oaks Drive, Suite 205
Sacramento, CA 95833
Phone: (916) 263-7800

Colorado Board of Nursing
1560 Broadway, Suite 880
Denver, CO 80202
Phone: (303) 894-2430

Idaho Board of Nursing
280 N. 8th Street, Suite 210
P.O. Box 83720
Boise, ID 83720
Phone: (208) 334-3110

Delaware Board of Nursing
861 Silver Lake Blvd
Cannon Building, Suite 203
Dover, DE 19904
Phone: (302) 739-4522

Florida Board of Nursing
4080 Woodcock Drive, Suite 202
Jacksonville, FL 32207
Phone: (904) 858-6940

**Georgia State Board of Licensed
Practical Nurses**
237 Coliseum Drive
Macon, GA 31217-3858
Phone: (912) 207-1300

Georgia Board of Nursing
237 Coliseum Drive
Macon, GA 31217-3858
Phone: (912) 207-1640

Guam Board of Nurse Examiners
P.O. Box 2816
1304 East Sunset Boulevard
Barrgada, GU 96913
Phone: (671) 475-0251

**Hawaii Board of Nursing
Professional & Vocational Licensing**
Division
P.O. Box 3469
Honolulu, HI 96801
Phone: (808) 586-3000

**Illinois Department of Professional
Regulation**
James R. Thompson Center
100 West Randolph, Suite 9-300
Chicago, IL 60601
Phone: (312) 814-2715

Indiana State Board of Nursing
Health Professions Bureau
402 W. Washington Street, Room W041
Indianapolis, IN 46204
Phone: (317) 232-2960

Iowa Board of Nursing
RiverPoint Business Park
400 S.W. 8th Street, Suite B
Des Moines, IA 50309-4685
Phone: (515) 281-3255

Kansas State Board of Nursing
Landon State Office Building
900 S.W. Jackson, Suite 551-S
Topeka, KS 66612
Phone: (785) 296-4929

Kentucky Board of Nursing
312 Whittington Parkway, Suite 300
Louisville, KY 40222
Phone: (502) 329-7000

**Louisiana State Board of Practical
Nurse Examiners**
3421 N. Causeway Boulevard, Suite 203
Metairie, LA 70002
Phone: (504) 838-5791

Louisiana State Board of Nursing
3510 N. Causeway Boulevard, Suite 501
Metairie, LA 70003
Phone: (504) 838-5332

Maine State Board of Nursing
158 State House Station
Augusta, ME 04333
Phone: (207) 287-1133

Maryland Board of Nursing
4140 Patterson Avenue
Baltimore, MD 21215
Phone: (410) 585-1900

**Massachusetts Board of Registration
in Nursing**
Commonwealth of Massachusetts
239 Causeway Street
Boston, MA 02114
Phone: (617) 727-9961

Michigan CIS/Office of Health Services
Ottawa Towers North
611 W. Ottawa, 4th Floor
Lansing, MI 48933
Phone: (517) 373-9102

Minnesota Board of Nursing
2829 University Avenue SE
Suite 500
Minneapolis, MN 55414
Phone: (612) 617-2270

Missouri State Board of Nursing
3605 Missouri Blvd.
P.O. Box 656
Jefferson City, MO 65102-0656
Phone: (573) 751-0681

Montana State Board of Nursing
301 South Park
Helena, MT 59620-0513
Phone: (406) 444-2071

**Commonwealth of Northern Mariana
Islands Board of Nurse Examiners**
Capitol Hill
Building 1336
Saipan, MP 96950
Phone: (670) 664-4810

**Nebraska Health and Human Services
Dept. of Regulation & Licensure**
Nursing Section
301 Centennial Mall South
Lincoln, NE 68509-4986
Phone: (402) 471-4376

New Hampshire Board of Nursing
P.O. Box 3898
78 Regional Drive, BLDG B
Concord, NH 03302
Phone: (603) 271-2323

New Jersey Board of Nursing
P.O. Box 45010
124 Halsey Street, 6th Floor
Newark, NJ 07101
Phone: (973) 504-6586

Mississippi Board of Nursing
1935 Lakeland Drive, Suite B
Jackson, MS 39216-5014
Phone: (601) 987-4188

New York State Board of Nursing
Education Bldg.
89 Washington Avenue
2nd Floor West Wing
Albany, NY 12234
Phone: (518) 474-3817, Ext. 120

North Carolina Board of Nursing
3724 National Drive, Suite 201
Raleigh, NC 27612
Phone: (919) 782-3211

North Dakota Board of Nursing
919 South 7th Street, Suite 504
Bismark, ND 58504
Phone: (701) 328-9777

Ohio Board of Nursing
17 South High Street, Suite 400
Columbus, OH 43215-3413
Phone: (614) 466-3947

Oklahoma Board of Nursing
2915 N. Classen Boulevard, Suite 524
Oklahoma City, OK 73106
Phone: (405) 962-1800

Oregon State Board of Nursing
800 NE Oregon Street, Box 25
Suite 465
Portland, OR 97232
Phone: (503) 731-4745

New Mexico Board of Nursing
4206 Louisiana Boulevard, NE, Suite A
Albuquerque, NM 87109
Phone: (505) 841-8340

Commonwealth of Puerto Rico
Board of Nurse Examiners
800 Roberto H. Todd Avenue
Room 202, Stop 18
Santurce, PR 00908
Phone: (787) 725-8161

**Rhode Island Board of Nurse
Registration and Nursing Education**
105 Cannon Building
Three Capitol Hill
Providence, RI 02908
Phone: (401) 222-5700

South Carolina State Board of Nursing
110 Centerview Drive, Suite 202
Columbia, SC 29210
Phone: (803) 896-4550

South Dakota Board of Nursing
4300 South Louise Ave., Suite C-1
Sioux Falls, SD 57106-3124
Phone: (605) 362-2760

Tennessee State Board of Nursing
426 Fifth Avenue North
1st Floor - Cordell Hull Building
Nashville, TN 37247
Phone: (615) 532-5166

Texas Board of Nurse Examiners
333 Guadalupe, Suite 3-460
Austin, TX 78701
Phone: (512) 305-7400

Pennsylvania State Board of Nursing
124 Pine Street
Harrisburg, PA 17101
Phone: (717) 783-7142

Utah State Board of Nursing
Heber M. Wells Bldg., 4th Floor
160 East 300 South
Salt Lake City, UT 84111
Phone: (801) 530-6628

Vermont State Board of Nursing
109 State Street
Montpelier, VT 05609-1106
Phone: (802) 828-2396

Virgin Islands Board of Nurse Licensure
Veterans Drive Station
St. Thomas, VI 00803
Phone: (340) 776-7397

Virginia Board of Nursing
6606 W. Broad Street, 4th Floor
Richmond, VA 23230
Phone: (804) 662-9909

Washington State Nursing Care Quality Assurance Commission
Department of Health
1300 Quince Street SE
Olympia, WA 98504-7864
Phone: (360) 236-4740

Texas Board of Vocational Nurse Examiners
William P. Hobby Building, Tower 3
333 Guadalupe Street, Suite 3-400
Austin, TX 78701
Phone: (512) 305-8100

West Virginia Board of Examiners for Licensed Practical Nurses
101 Dee Drive
Charleston, WV 25311
Phone: (304) 558-3572

West Virginia Board of Examiners for Registered Professional Nurses
101 Dee Drive
Charleston, WV 25311
Phone: (304) 558-3596

Wisconsin Department of Regulation and Licensing
1400 E. Washington Avenue
P.O. Box 8935
Madison, WI 53708
Phone: (608) 266-0145

Wyoming State Board of Nursing
2020 Carey Avenue, Suite 110
Cheyenne, WY 82002
Phone: (307) 777-7601

Nursing Program Accreditation

Contact either of the following organizations for a list of accredited nursing programs in the United States and its territories:

Commission on Collegiate Nursing Education
One Dupont Circle, NW, Suite 530
Washington, DC 20036
Phone: (202) 887-6791

National League for Nursing Accrediting Commission
61 Broadway, 33rd Floor
New York, NY 10006
Phone: (212) 363-5555, Ext. 153

Student Organizations

Chi Eta Phi Student Nurse Sorority
3029 13th Street, NW
Washington, DC 20009
Phone: (202) 232-3858

National Student Nurse Association
555 W. 57th Street
New York, NY 10019
Phone: (212) 581-2211

National Association for Practical Nurse Education and Service
1400 Spring St., Suite 330
Silver Spring, MD 20910
(301) 588-2491

Sigma Theta Tau International Nursing Honor Society
550 W. North Street
Indianapolis, IN 46202
Phone: (317) 634-8171

National Organization for Associate Degree Nursing
11250 Roger Bacon Drive, Suite 8
Reston, VA 20190-5202
Phone: (703) 437-4377

Financial Aid

Americorps Education Award
Corporation for National Service
1201 New York Avenue, NW
Washington, D.C. 20525
Phone: (202) 606-5000
AmeriCorps allows people of all ages and backgrounds to earn help paying for education in exchange for a year of volunteer service.

Federal Student Aid Information Center
P.O. Box 84
Washington, DC 20044
Phone: (800) 4-FED-AID
The Federal Student Aid information center is a clearinghouse of information on federal grants and loans for students.

U.S. Department of Veteran Affairs
Montgomery GI Bill Education Benefit
Phone: (888) 1-GI-BILL
This financial aid program is for United States Armed Forces veterans or members of the Selected Reserve, including the Army, Navy, Air Force, Marine Corps and Coast Guard Reserves, the Army National Guard and the Air Guard.

U.S. Public Health Service
Health Resources and Services Administration Bureau of Health Professions
5600 Fishers Lane
Rockville, Maryland 20857
The U.S. Public Health Service offers a variety of loans, scholarships, and loan repayment programs for students in the health professions.

Professional Associations

American Assembly for Men in Nursing
C/o NYSNA
11 Cornell Road
Latham, NY 12110-1499
Phone: (518) 782-9400, Ext. 346

American Licensed Practical Nurses Association
1090 Vermont Avenue, NW, Suite 1200
Washington, DC 20005
(202) 682-9000

American Nurses Association
600 Maryland Avenue, SW, Suite 100 West
Washington, DC 20024
Tel: (800) 274-4ANA

Asian & Pacific Islander Nurses Association
252 Silleck St.
Clifton, NJ. 07013
Phone: (718) 405-3354

National Alaska Native/American Indian Nurses Association
3702 S. Fife Street
Tacoma, WA 98409-7318
Phone: (888) 566-8773

National Association of Hispanic Nurses
1501 16th St., NW
Washington, DC 20036
Phone: (202) 387-2477

National Black Nurses Association
8630 Fenton Street, Suite 330
Silver Spring, MD 20910-3803
Phone: (301) 589-3200

National Federation of Licensed Practical Nurses
1418 Aversboro Road
Garner, SC 27529-4547
Phone: (919) 779-0046

National League for Nursing
61 Broadway, 33rd Floor
New York, NY 10006
Phone: (212) 363-5555 or
(800) 669-1656

Phillipine Nurses Association of America
151 Linda Vista Drive
Daly City, CA 94014
Phone: (415) 468-7995

For more great information, visit out our website. There you will find helpful articles that supplement this book, as well as a comprehensive listing of additional resources, including:

✦ Education and study skills.
✦ Distance learning.
✦ Grad school and advanced practice.
✦ NCLEX preparation.
✦ Certification in specialty areas.
✦ More sources of financial aid, grants and loans.
✦ Nursing journals and publications.
✦ Employment and career resources.

bandidobooks.com

References

American Psychological Association. (2001). *Publication Manual of the American Psychological Association* (5th Edition). Washington, DC: American Psychological Association.

Carey, K., Mee, C. (2001). *Nursing 2000 Salary Survey*. Retrieved June 10, 2001 from Springhouse Publishing Corporation's SpringNet at http://www.tnpj.com/content/nursing/0004/salsur04.htm

Heller, B., Oros, M., & Durney-Crowley, J. (1999). *The Future of Nursing Education: Ten Trends to Watch*. Retrieved May 10, 2001 from the National League for Nursing at http://www.nln.org/infotrends.htm

National Advisory Council on Nurse Education and Practice. (1996) *Report to the Secretary of the Department of Health and Human Services on the Basic Registered Nurse Workforce*. Washington, DC: U.S. Department of Health and Human Services, Health Resources and Services Administration, Bureau of Health Professions, Division of Nursing.

National Council of State Boards of Nursing. (1997). *NCLEX Examination Using CAT*. Chicago: National Council of State Boards of Nursing.

National Council of State Boards of Nursing. (2001). *NCLEX Candidate Examination Bulletin*. Chicago: National Council of State Boards of Nursing.

Opas, S. (1998). Pins and Pinning: The Traditions Continue. *RN Magazine, 12*, 49.

U.S. Department of Education. *Student Financial Assistance: Financial Aid from the U.S. Department of Education*. Retrieved May 31, 2001 from the U.S. Department of Education Federal Student Financial Aid Homepage at http://www.ed.gov/offices/OSFAP/Students

U.S. Department of Health and Human Services. (2001). *2000 National Sample Survey of Registered Nurses*. Rockville, MD: Division of Nursing, Bureau of Health Professions, Health Resources and Services Administration, U.S. Department of Health and Human Services.

U.S. Department of Labor. (2001). *Occupational Outlook Handbook*. Washington, DC: Division of Occupational Outlook, Bureau of Labor Statistics, U.S. Department of Labor.

Glossary

A

Accreditation - Official seal of approval by an accrediting organization indicating that a particular program has met specific, objective standards in the development and administration of its nursing education program.

Active Listening - The focused process of trying to understand what is being said or presented.

Active Reading - The process of reading with intent, defining ahead of time what concepts or information you are looking for to focus your attention.

Advanced Practice - Increased scope of practice for registered nurses resulting from specialized training and advanced education in a specific clinical area.

B

Bridge Programs - Accelerated degree completion programs for licensed nursing professionals. Available bridge program options include LPN to RN, RN to BSN and RN to MSN.

C

Career Ladder - An institutional program by which nurses are progressively promoted according to experience and/or education.

Care Plan - a written plan of action tailored specifically to a patient needs. It includes nursing diagnoses and patient assessment, nursing interventions to be used and expected outcomes.

Charting - Objectively and comprehensively documenting the condition and treatment of a patient.

Clinicals - Hands-on learning experiences in a variety of real clinical settings.

Common Law - Laws derived from principles or social mores rather than from rules and regulations. It consists of broad, interpretive principles based on reason, traditional justice and common sense

Confidentiality - A legal and ethical obligation to protect the privacy of healthcare consumers.

Critical Thinking - The ability to come to objective conclusions by evaluating all pertinent factors comprehensively. Applied knowledge and logical reasoning.

D

Differential Pay - Extra income added to base pay for such things as working the night shift, holidays, call-in and in some cases, for having specialty certification.

Distance Learning - Any type of educational program deliver outside of the normal classroom setting. This includes telecourses, internet courses and home-study programs.

Documentation - A written record of actions taken, events transpired and facts related to the condition of a patient. This includes patient history, assessments, interventions, medications given, updates on patient condition, etc.

F

Floating - A practice of many hospitals that requires nurses to occasionally work in other clinical areas to cover shortages.

H

Holistic Care - A method of providing care in which the whole person is considered during the assessment and treatment planning process. Physical, emotional, mental and spiritual needs are addressed.

L

Learning Objectives - Specific goals and outcomes of a particular course offering; what you should know after completing the course.

Licensure - A formal document of approval by the state board of nursing which is required to legally practice nursing. Licensure candidates must have graduated from an accredited nursing program and successfully passed the NCLEX exam.

Long Term Care Facility - Any healthcare facility designed to care for patients on a long-term basis, including nursing homes and rehabilitation centers.

N

NCLEX - National Council Licensure Examination; a standardized, national exam taken by nursing school graduates that is designed to measure and evaluate entry-level competencies in nursing.

Non-Traditional Student - Any student who does not fit the traditional profile of a college student. Non-traditional students may have independent financial status, spouses and/or children, or full-time careers. Also included are older adults, returning students and individuals pursuing a second career.

Nurse Practice Acts - Laws in each state that are instrumental in defining the scope of nursing practice. State boards of nursing oversee this statutory law.

Nurse Practitioner - A registered nurse with advanced education (a master's degree or advanced certification) and clinical training. Nurse Practitioners enjoy a wider scope of practice and increased autonomy.

Nursing Diagnosis - A statement of an actual or potential health problem that can be resolved through the assistance of nursing interventions.

Nursing Interventions - Therapeutic treatments administered by nurses to positively affect the health and well-being of their patients.

Nursing Process - A problem-solving process where data is gathered, analyzed and interpreted to assist in making clinical judgements, setting goals, establishing priorities and designing therapeutic nursing interventions.

 P

Pinning Ceremony - Traditional nursing school ceremony wherein graduating nurses received their nursing pin. Symbolic of initiation into the society of nurses.

Preceptor - An experienced nurse who acts as a mentor and supervisor to new nurses. Provides orientation, assigns work and remains available for ongoing support.

Prerequisite Courses - College-level courses which must be completed prior to entering a nursing program.

 S

Selective Admissions - An admissions policy that does not guarantee placement in a program even if all eligibility requirements have been met; eligible students compete for a limited number of openings.

 U

Universal Precautions - The term for infection control measures health care workers must follow to protect themselves and others from infectious disease. Universal precautions include hand washing, the use of protective gloves and other barrier protections, and following sterilization protocols.

Index

Notes

Notes

Notes

Notes

RESOURCES FOR NURSES

Nursing at Clinical Speed!

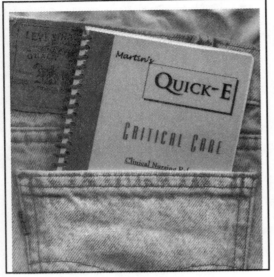

Get a Quick-E!

Martin's Quick-Es Clinical Nursing Reference
Handy pocket guides loaded with clinical facts and available right at the bedside. Plastic coil bound to enable ease of use, laminated for protection and they come with color index dividers to quickly access information when and where you need it! The book fits perfectly inside your lab or scrub pocket. We have even prepared each specialty title with *inspirational and entertaining quotes to brighten up the nursing day!* Specialty titles include Critical Care, ER, IV, Med-Surg, Assessment, Peds, OB, Spanish Guide and our new Quick-E Dysrhythmia (Cardiac Rhythm Interpretation). $19.95

***charlie brown* The Meanest Clipboard in Town!**
An ideal tool for the busy clinical setting. This handsomely crafted clipboard is loaded with often-needed clinical facts (lab values, assessment scales, dosage formulas, conversions etc.) imprinted on both sides! Plus, a built-in dual power calculator with big digit display! The perfect nursing tool for writing, reference and calculation.
$19.95

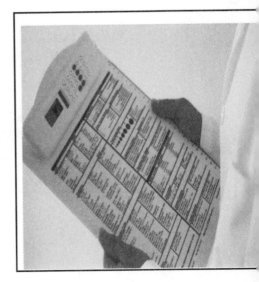

Over 50 lab values!

Available at www.bandidobooks.com or at a bookstore near you.

Happy Nursing!